THE
FATFIELD
Diet

The
FATFIELD
Diet
EAT MORE – WEIGH LESS

Sally Ann Voak

Michael O'Mara Books Limited

First published in Great Britain in 1991
by Michael O'Mara Books Limited

Revised edition first published in Great Britain in 1993
by Michael O'Mara Books Limited,
9 Lion Yard, Tremadoc Road, London SW4 7NQ

A CIP catalogue record for this book is available from the
British Library.

ISBN 1-85479-940-1

Designed by Mick Keates
Edited by Georgina Evans

Typeset by Florencetype Ltd, Kewstoke, Avon
Printed and bound by Cox & Wyman, Reading

CONTENTS

DEDICATION

To Toni, my terrific assistant and the best slimming counsellor I have ever worked with.

ACKNOWLEDGMENTS

A big thank you to Nerys Hughes, the Presenter of BBC's 'Bazaar'; Erica Griffiths, the Producer; Andy Smith, the Director; and Val Hudson, the Series Consultant. I'd also like to thank Susan Collins, the exercise class organiser, and, last but most important, the villagers of Fatfield, Tyne and Wear, England. Thank you all for making the Fatfield Experiment possible – and such fun too!

FOREWORD

by Dr Gaston L.S. Pawan, D.Sc. (Lond.), FRCPath.
Consultant in Human metabolism and Nutrition

Most overweight fat people would dearly love to be slim, not only because it is fashionable, but because it is well known that overweight increases the risk of heart disease, diabetes, arthritis and many other medical conditions. Physically and psychologically fat people are at a disadvantage. Their mobility, stamina and social life may be affected, and the problems they encounter in our figure- and fashion-conscious society can be formidable.

The question often asked is 'Why does a fat person become fat?' The usual answer given is 'He/she eats too much', and the solution to the problem is therefore 'Eat less and take more exercise' – hence the enormous number of 'slimming diets', exercise programmes and slimming gadgets available on the market. Yet, despite all these aids to slimming, success in losing weight satisfactorily and maintaining a normal bodyweight subsequently, is rare. It is a fact that many fat people may conscientiously follow a calorie-restricted diet for many weeks, often at great personal sacrifice, with some loss of bodyweight, but then on coming off the diet for various reasons, regain the lost weight. A most depressing experience!

Sally Ann Voak, the well-known journalist, author and broadcaster on health and beauty topics, has produced a completely new approach to the slimming problem. Her wide experience of slimmers, their problems and their diets, has led her to reject the usual approach to weight reduction based on the use of smaller meals to reduce calorie intake. Instead, she advocates the consumption of big, hearty, family-sized meals made up of wholesome healthy foods. She argues that in slimming, food should be fun. She shows how large, yet well-balanced, satisfying, calorie-controlled meals can produce steady and enjoyable weight loss. She explains how to relax, be motivated and, if necessary, be one's own counsellor. Simple exercises that are a pleasure to perform are described, and meal plans and recipes suitable for a variety of people, including vegetarians, are given.

I greatly enjoyed reading this book and enthusiastically recommend it. The sensible advice given by Sally Ann Voak should enable the overweight but otherwise healthy person slim successfully, achieve a normal bodyweight, and most importantly, avoid the weight regain so often experienced by slimmers.

Dr Gaston Pawan is Hon. Senior Lecturer, formerly Senior Lecturer, in Metabolism, Department of Medicine, The Middlesex Hospital and Medical School, London. He is Past Chairman of the Association for the Study of Obesity, and Past Chairman of the Board of Studies in Nutrition and Food Science, University of London.

CHAPTER ONE

WHY THIS DIET WORKS . . . WHEN OTHERS DON'T!

Congratulations! You have just joined the hundreds of thousands of successful slimmers who have already lost weight (and kept it off) on the Fatfield Diet. They are all agreed – it works! So you can now be absolutely certain of one thing: your dieting problems are almost over!

This is a promise that I have no hesitation in making for, since the first two Fatfield books appeared in 1991, I have been overwhelmed by the response from people who, after struggling with their weight problems for many years, have discovered that losing weight doesn't have to be a dreary process. In fact, it can be fun! I have had letters from thousands of people who read about the diet in *The Sun* newspaper, or saw the Fatfield villagers on the BBC-TV programme 'Bazaar'.

Many of them had become stuck on the dieting 'treadmill' of alternate bingeing and crash-dieting. But once they tried the Fatfield Diet, they found that getting slim – and even more important *staying* slim – is far easier than they could ever have imagined possible.

They have also found to their amazement that you really can 'eat more and weigh less', and re-train your eating habits so that you no longer crave the high-fat, high-sugar foods that make the pounds pile on. So for many of these slimmers, eating the Fatfield way has become more than just a diet – it's become a way of life.

Here are extracts from just a few of the letters I've received:

Julianne Whiteley from Letchworth, Herts wrote: 'I am just writing to thank you from the bottom of my heart for giving me the inspiration to lose the excess weight I've been carrying since I was 16. I began the Fatfield Steady Weight Loss Diet weighing over 11 stone, and easily slimmed down to 9 stone 12lb in just a few months. My statistics have changed from 40D–40–40 to 34C–25–35. I'm a size 10 for the first time in my life. I have tried slimming programmes before, with very limited success. Your advice and diets beat all the rest!'

Bruce Glasser from Redbourne, Herts says: 'I lost 3 stone in eight months and felt wonderful. I wasn't hungry at all and felt really healthy and well. What's more, I've maintained my weight-loss for over a year. I really recommend the diet – it's great.'

Mary Thurston, from Ipswich, Suffolk wrote: 'I read both Fatfield books with great enjoyment. I lost 2½ stone in six months and now weigh 8 stone 4lb. I loved the recipes and use them all the time.'

Yvette Bainbridge, from Washington, Tyne and Wear, wrote: 'I weighed 16½ stone when I started the diet. I am now down to 12 stone and feel like a different person. Since learning to eat the Fatfield way, I have totally changed my shopping and cooking habits. My five little daughters are also benefitting from the healthier way of eating. I was surprised at how inexpensive foods are, too. There is certainly no need to spend a lot to slim successfully. And your claim that slimmers should eat more to weigh less really is true! Thank you.'

Elizabeth Montgomery from Carlisle wrote: 'After seeing your Fatfield villagers on the BBC 'Bazaar' programme, I decided that if they could lose weight, I could do it too! I rushed out and bought your book and I can honestly say that it has changed my life.

'When I started the diet I was over 14 stone and feeling extremely miserable. Despite efforts to lose weight, the pounds had piled on over the years, and, at 45, I felt that I had left it too late to slim. But, not a bit of it! The first week I lost 6lb, and I then shed 2 or 3lb a week until I reached 10 stone. I have maintained that weight for almost six months and feel very confident that my tubby days are over.'

Jim Elliott from Birmingham says: 'If this is a slimming diet, I am astounded! I followed the Boozers' Plan because I do enjoy a pint or two. Once I'd got used to eating differently, I found it very simple to follow. I lost 3 stone in just two months and my wife lost 2 stone. We are delighted.'

All these slimmers have one thing in common: they had all tried dieting before with very little success. Either they had lost weight and put it back on again, or the diet had been hopeless from the word 'go'.

By following the Fatfield Diet, they gave their health a valuable boost, improved their skin, hair, and general vitality – oh yes, and they lost a lot of weight as well!

They, and you, are following in the footsteps of an extremely demanding panel of slimmers: the people of Fatfield, Tyne and Wear, England. These are the people who proved to me that you can slim without suffering, without spending a fortune, and without putting yourself on a potentially disastrous 'yo-yo' cycle of losing and gaining weight.

What's more, you can sit down to large, satisfying, family-size meals with friends and loved ones while the pounds drop off. There is no need to cook special meals or eat different foods from everyone else. This is important because, time and time again, slimmers give up the fight when diet meals are boring, too small or even replaced altogether by less-than-appetising drinks. The problem with all these diets is that at some point you have to come off them and wean yourself back onto normal foods. Frankly, it just isn't necessary to give up normal foods in the first place. The supermarkets now have such a wide variety of choice and give such excellent information on packs that you can buy everything you need at your usual shopping venue.

So, even if you normally start a slimming programme on Monday, and give up on Tuesday, this is one plan you will stick to . . . not just painlessly, but with relish!

FOOD IS FUN

The Fatfield Diet is different from many other diets which seem to assume that slimmers want to suffer while they lose pounds. It works on the wicked principle that eating is life's second greatest pleasure. (No prizes for guessing what is life's top pleasure!) Food should be enjoyed, savoured and eaten with delicious relish. Every meal should be a feast – from the sandwich you nibble alone at lunchtime to the fabulous dinner you sit down to at Christmas or on some other special occasion. Food is comforting. Food is sexy. Food is indulgent. Food is sensual. Food is wonderful!

Luckily, current nutritional thinking encourages a type of eating that goes along with these refreshingly greedy principles. Over the last few years, scientists and doctors have come up with a set of sensible guidelines which help you to eat more and weigh less. Although nutrition is still a young science which is evolving all the time, these ideas will stick around for many years because they have been proved to be healthy, thanks to a number of controlled studies.

The main guidelines laid down by the scientists are that we should all cut back on fat and sugar, and increase the amount of fibre in our diet. It is particularly important to cut back on fat, as an excessive intake of fat has been linked to heart disease so convincingly that the vast majority of doctors now accept this as fact. Sadly, people in this country still get an amazing 40 per cent of their daily calories from fat, which is why we have one of the highest incidences of heart disease in the world. However, it must be noted that *some* fat is essential for good health – so if you are tempted to follow a diet which recommends cutting out fat altogether, beware!

Sugar is another 'baddie' because it provides huge amounts of calories with no other nutrients. We eat approximately 2lb of sugar per person every week in Britain – most of it the 'hidden' kind in processed foods, biscuits and confectionery. That's the equivalent of 3500 calories, which is enough for a whole day's meals for a man in a strenuous job. So, it is obvious that many overweight people can blame their 'sweet tooth' habit for at least some of their slimming problems. It makes sense, therefore, to cut down on both kinds of sugar – in your tea and in foods. On the Fatfield Diet, you do just that but in such a way that you never ever feel deprived of your sugar 'fix'.

Fibre, in fruits, vegetables, pulses like peas and beans, and grains, is a 'goodie' because it helps prevent diseases such as bowel cancer, diverticulitis, diabetes and heart disease. Foods containing plenty of fibre also have the advantage of being extremely filling, so they figure strongly in the Fatfield Diet.

But, believe me, you won't have to go without meals like sausages and mash, burgers and chips. You certainly won't be asked to give up delicious puddings, sweet snacks and treats, and you will not be eating so many fibre-rich baked beans that your friends will wonder if you are following the F..tfield Diet!

To help you turn meal times into the special occasions they should be, we have devised some brand new recipes especially for this new edition which will fit into your lifestyle. All the recipes in the book are very easy to make and the ingredients are available from your supermarket. There are soups and starters, supper dishes, picnic and barbecue treats, wicked desserts and tasty snacks. Each recipe can be adapted to feed any number of people, from a large family to a single person. Every dish is guaranteed to fill you up. On the Fatfield diet, every meal is a whopping great meal!

HOW TO FOLLOW THE DIET

Please do *not* start the diet until you have read the whole book, from cover to cover. It will help your own slimming campaign to read all about the problems, occasional disasters and triumphs of our Fatfield guinea-pigs. The chapters on coping with your slimming campaign and finding motivation will provide invaluable inspiration. The exercise section will help you tone up while the pounds drop off. If the very thought of working out makes you feel limp and tired, don't worry. The Fatfield exercises are the easiest you have ever tackled. The only jogging you are asked to do is around the house, the only aerobics exercises are in a swimming pool so you do not feel the pain (or risk injuring yourself), and every work-out takes 20 minutes, or even less.

At the end of the book is a special section. Here there is a Calorie Guide to branded foods which I recommend for Fatfield slimmers. These have been selected for their nutritional value and appetite-appeal. In other words, they are tummy-filling, delicious and a useful addition to your shopping list. What's more, they have all been tested by a special panel of Fatfield food tasters and given top marks for scrumptiousness and value.

You will also find a Food Diary which I want you to fill in each day for a week, recording your meal intake, details of snacks, and how you coped with the diet. There is an address on page 108 where you can write with any problems you may have, and receive *free* advice from the Fatfield Diet slimming counsellors. If you want to be put in touch with a Slim Pal, for mutual support, full details are given too.

The most important thing of all is the Fatfield Charter. All slimmers should sign this before starting the diet. It is up to you whether you reveal your slimming ambitions to your family or friends. If you do decide to do this, pin the Charter on the kitchen wall for everyone to see. If you prefer to be a secret slimmer, keep the charter hidden away in a drawer, but DO sign it, as a constant reminder of your vow to stick to the plan.

Now, try the quiz below. It's fun, and also deadly serious, because it will help you to pinpoint approximately how many calories you are consuming right now. You could be surprised. Don't cheat!

HOW MUCH DO YOU REALLY EAT?

1. Which of these describes most closely your usual weekday breakfast meal? (Tick *one*)
    a) Cereal, milk, slice of toast and marmalade, tea or coffee
    b) Toast and a cup of tea or coffee
    c) Egg, bacon, sausage, beans, tea
    d) Nothing at all, or just a beverage

2. Which of these is most like your weekday lunch? (Tick *one*)
    a) Burger and chips
    b) Cooked meal in canteen or at home, such as chop and vegetables, pudding to follow
    c) Sandwiches and fruit or yogurt
    d) Sandwiches and crisps
    e) Pub lunch
    f) Chinese or Indian takeaway
    g) Salad with cheese, meat or fish

3. Which of these is most like your supper meal?
    a) Meat or fish and selection of vegetables
    b) Three course meal of soup, fish or meat, pudding
    c) Takeaway meal of fish and chips, Chinese, Indian, pizza
    d) Frozen ready-meal from supermarket
    e) Slimmer's ready-meal
    f) Snack meal: beans or egg on toast

4. Which of these between-meals snacks and confectionary items do you eat? (Tick them *all* – no cheating!)

8

a) About one packet of biscuits a day
b) Up to four biscuits a day
c) One or two bars of chocolate
d) A few sweets
e) A couple of slices of bread or toast and butter
f) A scoop of icecream or iced lolly
g) Bag of chips
h) Slice of pizza

5. What is your daily alcohol consumption? (One unit is the equivalent of half a pint of beer or lager OR one pub measure short drink with a mixer, OR one glass of wine)
   a) 2 units, or less
   b) 2–4 units
   c) 4–6 units
   d) 6–8 units

6. What other drinks do you consume?
   a) Tea or coffee with milk and sugar – 2 or 3 cups daily
   b) Tea or coffee without sugar – 2 or 3 cups daily
   c) Tea or coffee with milk and sugar – 3–6 cups daily
   d) Tea or coffee without sugar – 3–6 cups daily
   e) Tea or coffee without milk and sugar
   f) Canned fizzy drinks – 1 or 2
   g) Canned fizzy drinks – 2–4 daily

7. How much fruit do you eat?
   a) 1 piece daily (eg. apple, orange, pear, grapefruit, slice of melon)
   b) 2 pieces daily
   c) 3 pieces daily

8. What are the main cooking methods used in your home? (Tick *one*)
   a) Lots of fry-ups using fat or oil
   b) Mainly grilling or roasting with a little fat added
   c) Grilling, steaming, baking – no fat added

NOW ADD UP YOUR SCORE

1. a) 250   b) 100   c) 400   d) 0
2. a) 650   b) 550   c) 500   d) 500   e) 700
   f) 1000   g) 300
3. a) 450   b) 650   c) 1000   d) 550   e) 300
   f) 350
4. a) 800   b) 350   c) 500   d) 350   e) 300
   f) 100   g) 350   h) 400
5. a) 200   b) 400   c) 600   d) 800
6. a) 150   b) 60   c) 250   d) 0   e) 120
   f) 140   g) 350
7. a) 50   b) 100   c) 150
8. a) 150   b) 100   c) 0

The total will tell you, approximately, how many calories you are consuming each day. The average woman burns up around 2000 calories a day, and the average man between 2500–3000 calories.

It is very easy to exceed this total. For instance, if, on our quiz, you have ticked 1a, 2b, 3c, 4d, 5a, 6a, 7a and 8b your daily calorie total is just over 2500. This is fine if you are a man who wants to stay the same weight, but disastrous if you are a woman who wants to lose weight. In fact, with a pound of body weight being roughly equivalent to 3500 calories, you are probably putting on weight at the rate of around 1lb a week. Which might not sound much, but adds up to nearly 4 stone a year!

But, I promise you that is the very last sum you have to do. On the Fatfield Diet I have done all the sums for you. You will be cutting calories safely and easily while adding bulk and filling-power to your meals.

NOW GET RID OF GUILT

After completing the quiz above, you are probably feeling riddled with guilt about the amount you are eating and drinking.

Before you start reading more about the diet that is going to work for you, I want you to do something very difficult: stop feeling guilty – right now!

In twenty years of slimming counselling, my assistants and I have helped thousands of people to reach their ideal weight. The biggest hurdle we have had to overcome has been guilt. Guilt is time-wasting, destructive and fattening. It makes slimmers worry about their ability to stick to a diet, about being selfish while they are on the diet, and also about giving in during moments of extreme temptation. Every overweight person I have ever counselled – from politicians to pop singers – has felt guilty about their eating habits, particularly about their cravings for big, satisfying meals. In many cases, the guilt feelings are so strong that they make slimmers turn to the wrong kinds of food for comfort, which generates more guilt, and so on.

Why all this guilt? For my own post-war generation, guilt is often generated by our memories of childhood meals where food was so precious that every scrap had to be consumed. Hearty, inexpensive high-fat dishes like bread and dripping, mutton stew and roly-poly pudding were often on the menu, and woe betide the child who didn't leave a clean plate. Many of the middle-aged slimmers I work with today feel they are letting their parents down if they don't eat up enormous meals every day! It

11

seems wicked to sit down to a lettuce leaf and some cottage cheese when good food is available. Luckily, on the Fatfield Diet, you never, ever sit down to such a meagre meal: quite the opposite.

Younger slimmers have grown up in a confused world; they are constantly exposed to magazine articles, television programmes and news reports about the dangers of overeating, yet they are expected to ignore the temptations around them. These days, every high street has a wide range of fast-food restaurants and takeaways to choose from. Every supermarket has such a huge selection of tempting goodies that they make you long for an orgy of doughnuts, pasties and meat pies. Although most of them now give good nutritional information in special leaflets or on packets, they still stock high-fat foods, and some still tempt adults and, even worse, children with confectionery displays at check-outs. No wonder one of my slimmers was so overcome with guilt after a supermarket car-park feast of sausage rolls that she burst into tears of shame!

So, what do you do? First, try to accept that you are a victim of childhood conditioning (we all are!) and very likely to be exposed to temptation every single day of your life. You are not a saint. So, some days, you may fail. So what? You can always make up for it the day after. There is no need to feel guilty, to shed tears or to blame yourself for your 'weakness'. You are not weak, just vulnerable. In any case, you will reduce the chances of failure considerably because you are on the Fatfield Diet.

I know this to be true because I follow it myself! It is the only diet that truly fits into my family life, satisfies my craving for large, hearty meals, and yet allows me to stay slim. I now weigh 8 stone 12lb, exactly the same as when I married nearly 30 years ago, and over a stone less than I weighed as a teenager.

What's more, I don't feel guilty about my two pints of Guinness a day, my occasional desire for chocolate, or my lust for French cooking. On the Fatfield Diet, I can have them all!

CHAPTER TWO

THE FATFIELD EXPERIMENT

I first started writing about slimming back in 1974. Then, high-protein diets were frequently recommended. Doctors advised their overweight patients to stop eating bread and potatoes (incredibly, some still do) and eat plenty of steaks, fatty roasts and hard-boiled eggs. Not surprisingly, people developed bad breath, became constipated and got very bored when trying to slim down. In those days it was fashionable for women to have an ultra-thin 'Twiggy'-like body. Many became ill in their quest to achieve the perfect shape.

Strange theories abounded: people latched onto any crazy eating plan that sounded as though it might work. They stuffed themselves with bananas and milk or ate a whole grapefruit without sugar before every meal, or even made themselves sick and messed up their metabolism by taking appetite-suppressing drugs.

At around that time, books and specialist magazines started to appear which examined the whole subject of losing weight in much more detail. Scientists discovered that we need more fibre in our diet, the links between high fat consumption and heart disease were explored, and the importance of trace elements and enzymes was revealed. A much healthier approach to dieting was encouraged. At

14

the same time, slimming clubs started to open up. Each club had its own diet plan with group leaders (usually successful slimmers themselves) to help members to put it into action. The club method of slimming worked well, and continues to do so. However, some overweight people have found that the often rigid approach can be off-putting and, of course, the club's standard does depend to a very great extent on the leader's ability to inspire his or her members.

While slimming publications and clubs educated overweight people about a healthier approach to dieting, there were also some interesting new ideas on treating the psychological problems associated with obesity. At lectures and seminars, psychologists expounded their views on the 'new' ways to help people to slim successfully. We were told that 'comfort eating' was a peculiarly feminine problem, and could only be solved if women became more assertive; dieting was suddenly a dirty word! Then, behaviour therapy became popular. We were told that meals must be eaten at the right time, in the correct environment and food must be chewed a certain number of times with a long pause between mouthfuls. It was all useful stuff, although sometimes taken to extremes and often impractical. These days, most men would take exception to being told that scoffing comfort foods is just a female problem!

As a reporter, I informed my readers about *all* of these fascinating things. But they still wrote to me in their thousands wanting the perfect diet, and they were still willing to try almost anything in the vain hope that, this time, they had found it.

I endeavoured to make sure that the tips I passed on didn't give them any false hopes by trying out all the newest diets and slimming theories on volunteers. Instead of picking as my 'guinea pigs' members of slimming clubs who are already highly motivated to slim, I prefer to work with individuals or groups of people who find it very difficult to follow a diet because of the job they do, their lifestyle, or their environment. Among the well-known individuals I have helped to slim are MP Emma Nicholson (who lost 20lb), Lord Prior (who lost 1½ stone to raise money for Great Ormond Street Children's Hospital), comedian Frank Carson (he shed 3 stone), presenter Shane Richie (he needed to lose a stone for flying sequences in *Peter Pan*) and 'Birds of a Feather' star, Linda Robson (she trimmed off a stone).

My latest slimming 'star' is wonderful Marion Shergold, mother of brave cancer sufferer Craig Shergold – the boy who raised over a million pounds for research by setting a record for the number of get-well cards he received. Marion put on weight when she was worried sick about Craig and neglecting her own diet. Like any mother, she put her child first, but she didn't realise that her own health was suffering too. Now she eats more than ever before, looks wonderful, and has lost over 5 stone in just over a year.

Four years ago, I organised the first of my group slim-ins for *The Sun*. We helped 100 villagers from Broadbottom, near Manchester, to shed 100 stone in a month to raise cash for their annual carnival. The villagers love their food – and drink. So it seemed rather dangerous to run the weekly weigh-in at the local pub. In fact that turned out to be a splendid idea, as everyone could celebrate their weight-loss afterwards using up the generous alcohol allowance I gave them.

The Broadbottom experience convinced me that eating large meals while you slim down really does work. So I enlisted two more groups of people to help prove the theory once and for all. Eighty stallholders at Tommy-field's Market, Oldham, were trimmed into shape, and a group of workers at Fremlin's Brewery in Maidstone, Kent, also lost weight. This time, 30 slimmers lost 30 stone between them in just six weeks.

Then the BBC asked me to help slim people working in jobs where it is particularly difficult to stay trim, for the popular daytime programme, 'Bazaar'. The programme, now in its fifth series, is screened twice weekly from July to September, and is packed with brilliant ideas and tips on everything from DIY to cooking. I found two traffic police-men who were expanding rapidly, and two lorry drivers who were putting on weight fast. All four were 'comfort' eating because of the stressful nature of their jobs. In both cases, I provided a diet plan that fitted in with their lifestyles, including snacks to eat on the road and comfort-ing meals to eat at home. Once more, the one thing that made them all stick to the diet was that they ate so much food.

Two years ago, I suggested to 'Bazaar's producer, Erica Griffiths, that we should try to help a whole commu-nity of people to slim down and get fit. The idea was to help them re-train their eating habits over the full six months that the series then ran, from January to June 1991. Little did we know that the villagers of Fatfield, Tyne and Wear, England would *still* be slimming away two years later, and would lose nearly two *tons* of weight between them! In fact, after being featured in three 'Bazaar' series and in *The Sun* newspaper, the village is so famous that tourists go there to sightsee, and meet the people who found out how to slim so painlessly!

Fatfield proved to be a wonderful choice for a health experiment. It is a gorgeous little village, nestling on the banks of the River Wear, about 15 miles from the port of

Sunderland, close to the modern town of Washington, and around 8 miles from Newcastle-upon-Tyne. Once a flourishing mining village, it is now largely residential with just three public houses, a couple of churches, a village school and two busy taxi firms.

Back in the seventeenth century it was a bustling industrial centre with a corn mill, an iron foundry and thriving businesses making coal tar, lamp black and coke. Flat-bottomed boats based at Fatfield brought the coal down the river to Sunderland for transportation to London. The keelmen who piloted the boats were such a huge, terrifying bunch that pressgangs looking for naval recruits avoided the area. By all accounts, the Fatfield people had a very hard life. The miners worked long hours in a dirty, dangerous job. Their wives worked equally hard, cooking hot meals throughout the day, and washing their men's dust-covered clothes. Most households included several men working at the pit, on different shifts, so the poor lady of the house had to get up at all hours, and put meals on the table throughout the day. It is not surprising that the people had huge appetites, filling up on local specialities like pies, dumplings, best beef, mutton, kneaded cakes and black pudding. You can still see these traditional dishes being made at the famous Beamish Museum near Fatfield.

The Fatfielders still have huge appetites. They can shop at the excellent supermarkets in Washington, or buy from local speciality shops. Pies, pasties and dumplings are still just as popular as they were a hundred years ago. In addition, villagers eat the modern foods which so often contribute to weight problems: chips, pizzas, Chinese and Indian takeaways, cakes and confectionery.

On my first visit to Fatfield, I had lunch at the attractive Riverside Inn and was astonished by the size of the meal. My huge, oval plate was piled high with a vast piece of fish in batter, an enormous mound of chips and an outsize portion of mushy peas, a local speciality made with dried peas flavoured with sugar. The calorie count of this plateful was around 1000, a lot for one meal. As I ploughed my way through it (without guilt!), I realised that if the eating programme succeeded here it would succeed anywhere!

Within a few months of our first meeting in January 1991, over 50 Fatfield villagers had lost more than 50 stone in weight. By summer, the weight-loss had soared to half a ton, and by the start of the next 'Bazaar' series in 1992, they had shed a whole ton of weight.

The Fatfielders now meet regularly each Wednesday at the Biddick Inn on the banks of the River Wear. Many of our members also work out with local fitness expert Susan Collins. Sue teaches at the Washington Leisure Centre. We start our very overweight slimmers off with some gentle aquafit exercises (in water), and they gradually progress to low-impact aerobics and even circuit training as the weight drops off. Many of our members have completely reshaped their bodies, and changed their lives, too: pretty Vera Churnside has lost 3 stone, and has just completed a business studies and computer technology course. Glamorous gran, Linda Philpott, has shed 2½ stone and become the star of the local aerobics group. Lovely Julie Robson has trimmed away 5 stone and is now a cover girl (see the cover of this book!)

The project has expanded too. We now run a separate group at another pub, The Happy Wanderer at Framwellgate Moor, near Durham. This pub has excellent food, too, with lots of Fatfield dishes on the menu. No doubt there will be more Fatfield Slimming Pubs in the future!

So, the diet now has an excellent track record of success. In the next chapter, you will find out just how you can be part of this success. Go for it!

CHAPTER THREE

HEARTY EATING IS HEALTHY EATING

Are you fed up with being told that you should eat less to be healthy? Relax. For once in your life, you are about to be told that you probably do not eat *enough*.

Mealtimes are, on the whole, enjoyable occasions and any diet plan which makes you *stop* enjoying your food should be avoided. If you have ever tried to slim down and failed miserably because you stopped looking forward to your meals, you will know what I mean. That awful, depressing feeling which comes over you when you know that your family will be sitting down to a delicious Shepherd's Pie, vegetables and a big pudding, while you fiddle around with a boring salad, is familiar to most people. You kid yourself that the sacrifice will be worthwhile when you are able, at last, to struggle into a size 12 dress, or if you are a man buy a pair of 34-inch-waist trousers. Sadly, you will probably start to expand again once you go back to eating normally.

The body is like a car: it needs regular injections of 'fuel', that is food, to run smoothly and efficiently. That means we should eat three times a day, or even more. We use breakfast, lunch and supper as a means of breaking up the day as well as replenishing our tummies. For most of us, these meals are associated with social activities as well as putting food into our mouths. You may not feel that you

20

are particularly social at breakfast, but you probably eat the first meal of the day (if you do bother to eat it) while you talk to your family, scan the papers or open the post. At lunchtime perhaps you chat to work colleagues or listen to the radio. In the evening, you probably eat supper while you talk through the day with your partner, or watch television. In each case, you have combined eating with another activity, which makes it doubly important in your life. To my mind this is as it should be.

But, if eating is good for us, why is around 50 per cent of the population overweight? The answer lies in what we eat. Consider these two menus, eaten by one of our Fatfield slimmers, a lady in her mid-thirties with two children and a part-time job. The first menu is a typical example of the food eaten during a working day before she started following the Fatfield Diet. The second is very similar to the kind of daily menu she enjoys today. As you can see she is now eating *more* than she was before.

BEFORE DIETING

Breakfast: cup of tea with full-cream milk and 2 teaspoons of sugar

Mid-Morning: 4 digestive biscuits, cup of coffee with full-cream milk and 2 teaspoons of sugar

Lunch: Beefburger and chips, fizzy drink

Mid-Afternoon: slice of chocolate cake, cup of tea with full-cream milk and 2 teaspoons of sugar

Supper: lamb chop, chips, grilled tomatoes, individual fruit pie, $^1/_2$ pint of lager or a glass of wine, cup of tea with full-cream milk and 2 teaspoons of sugar

This menu does not appear to be excessively heavy. For a start, the lady had no breakfast and a fairly light supper. She experienced hunger pangs throughout the day, particularly just before lunch, and during the evening while watching television. She had tried to slim in the past by cutting out biscuits and chips, but somehow could never stick to this. The foods on the menu contain about 115 grams of fat, only 10 grams of fibre and approximately 2500 calories.

ON THE FATFIELD DIET

Breakfast: 1 cup of tea with skimmed milk and sweetener, 1 slice of wholemeal toast topped with 2 tablespoons baked beans, grilled tomatoes

Mid-Morning: 1 pear, 2 crispbreads topped with low-fat cheese, 1 cup of coffee with skimmed milk and sweetener

Lunch: 1 mug of slimmer's soup, large wholemeal sandwich with filling of salad, cold cooked chicken, 1 pear, 1 glass of mineral water

Mid-Afternoon: 1 low-calorie fruit yogurt, 1 cup of tea with skimmed milk and sweetener

Supper: Portion of Fatfield Shepherd's Pie (*see* recipe, page 139), green beans, carrots, braised onion, baked apple stuffed with a few raisins, $1/2$ pint of lager or a glass of wine, cup of tea with skimmed milk and sweetener

When she was shown this menu, our slimmer protested that she would never be able to eat all the foods listed. However, she soon became used to the additional bulk, and the weight simply dropped off. She lost 20lb in two months comfortably without being hungry or miserable. The foods on the menu contain about 60 grams of fat, 56 grams of fibre and approximately 1300 calories.

As you can see, the second menu is much lower in calories than the first. It also contains more fibre and less fat. With a calorie saving of around 1200 daily, this slimmer was able to lose weight easily, despite eating more food, in terms of bulk, than she had ever eaten in her life!

WHY CALORIES COUNT

Never believe any diet plan that tells you that you do not need to worry about calories. Sorry, folks, but I am afraid this is a big myth! Diets that tell you to eat certain foods at certain times of day, diets that preach that 'unlimited' amounts of meat and eggs will slim you down, diets that suggest alternating fruity days with indulgent days – they are *all* doomed to failure unless the basic sum (i.e. calorie intake must be *less* than calorie expenditure to produce weight-loss) is followed.

Especially dangerous are diets that consist of menus which do not specify exactly how much to eat. The authors are hoping that you will be so sick of a certain food, such as meat, that you will keep the amount to within sensible limits. In my work with thousands of slimmers, I know that nutritionists and dieticians often severely underestimate the ability of overweight people to consume huge amounts. While an 'average' 3oz (75g) portion of say, ham, only contains about 150 calories, some slimmers' ideas of an 'average' amount may be a half-pound of ham, thus adding 400 calories to the daily total. The *only* foods that you can eat freely on any diet (including this one – see page 35 for details) are leafy greens and salad vegetables which contain so few calories that you would have to stuff yourself silly to achieve a weight-gain if they were your only source of calories. The only drink that you can consume freely is water (which contains no calories at all). Diet soft drinks, black coffee and tea can, in theory, also be consumed freely, but too much of any of these is bad for your health and can affect, adversely, the success of your diet. Therefore, we do limit them on the Fatfield Diet.

So what is a calorie? The scientific definition is that it is the amount of energy needed to increase the temperature of 1 gram of water by 1 degree Centigrade. Sometimes, you see calories referred to as kilocalories. This is a more accurate name, really, because the kind of calories we are talking about would raise the temperature of 1 kilogram (i.e. nearly 2 pints) of water by 1 degree Centigrade.

If all that sounds like mumbo jumbo to you, don't worry. A much easier way of imagining what calories are is to think of them as, simply, units of energy supplied by the nutrients contained in food. The number of calories contained in a food depends on the kind of food it is. For instance, 1 gram of carbohydrate (in potatoes, bread, cereals, fruit) produces about 3.75 calories; 1 gram of fat (butter, lard, cooking oil, fat in meat) produces about 9 calories; 1 gram of protein (meat, eggs, fish) produces 4 calories and 1 gram of alcohol produces 7 calories. If you are measuring your food in ounces (as most people in the United Kingdom still are!), all you need to do is think of 100 grams as approximately 4 ounces. As you can see, foods which are high in fat produce the most calories, but 'booze' is pretty high too.

We 'spend' just over 1 calorie a minute merely to stay alive. That is, to maintain bodily functions such as breathing and digesting food. Once we do anything, sitting, walking, sleeping, exercising, the calorie expenditure increases accordingly. Of course, the total energy expended on any task depends not only upon the work involved but also upon the amount of energy the individual puts into it.

For instance, a very overweight person may be sluggish and droopy, even when performing simple tasks like walking around the house. On the other hand, they will certainly need to use up extra energy simply to move their bulk around from place to place.

So, calorie expenditure is a very individual thing, varying from person to person, depending on their lifestyle, weight, activities, and the amount of enthusiasm they put into them. Our daily calorie expenditure is also affected by some forms of medication (such as steroids and tranquillizers, which can make body metabolism and therefore energy expenditure sluggish), by changes in lifestyle (such as a change of job), by pregnancy and illness, smoking (and giving it up!) and even by emotional things like worry and falling in love.

However, the experts who have to decide what constitutes a healthy diet have given us guidelines to help us work out how many calories we need. As a rough guide, a woman in a sedentary job needs only around 2000 calories daily, a man around 2500.

This means that the vast majority of people can lose weight satisfactorily on 1500 calories daily. Certainly, women who are 2 or 3 stone overweight and most men should have no difficulty in shedding weight on a 1500 calorie diet. Women who have less weight to lose can do so very nicely on around 1200–1300 calories daily. *Unless* they have been putting their body into what we in the trade call 'starvation mode'.

This can happen when you have been following a diet that is very low in calories – usually *too* low. Since the human body is incredibly adaptable, it becomes used to this amount of nourishment each day. Your body 'decides' that you have probably been marooned in the desert with just starvation rations, or sent on a mission to the moon which has overshot, and food is running out. So, when you suddenly increase your calorie intake, your body conserves energy like crazy, laying down fat stores in case you are not rescued from the desert, or that mission to the moon. The best way to deal with this situation is to 'rev up' your metabolism by eating little and often, gradually increasing calories to a more sensible level, and stepping up exercise at the same time. The Fatfield Diet has a special plan for people who are experiencing this problem, which also works very well if you are stuck on a dieting 'plateau', where weight simply refuses to budge. If you have this difficulty check it out on page 85.

So, if calories matter so much, surely it is a good idea to throw away diet books, buy a good calorie counter and work out your own menus? Sorry, but NO! The problem here is that it can be all too tempting to 'spend' your daily calorie allowance on foods that you enjoy but do not do you much good. You then check your calorie total at lunchtime and find, to your horror, that you have already consumed 1500 calories in biscuits, sweets and soft drinks. There is nothing left for supper. Even if you have sufficient will-power and nutritional know-how to plan sensible meals, it is very fiddly indeed to work out exactly how many calories they contain, and you could fool yourself by leaving out things like cooking oil, drinks, and nibbles.

What *is* a good idea, is to start becoming 'calorie aware'. That is, to be canny enough to know which foods are high in calories and which are low. It means you should start looking at branded foods in supermarkets (many – although not enough – now give calorie values on the packaging), and checking out the list of Favourite Fatfield Foods on page 159. Our Fatfield slimmers have been doing some supermarket spot-checking and food-tasting themselves, and we have compiled a list of their favourite low-calorie buys. They have all been tested by our slimming team, and rated tops for value, taste and slim-power.

A final note on calories: there are very few people indeed who will not lose weight on a calorie-controlled diet. If you think you are one of these few, talk to your doctor before trying this, or any other diet. But first, keep a food diary for a week (*see* page 163), to make absolutely sure that you are not kidding yourself, and wasting your doctor's time.

FAT MAKES YOU FAT

Imagine a greasy, glutinous globule of fat. It is shiny, runny and looks absolutely disgusting as it disappears down the drain. It looks equally disgusting, hard and white, as it floats obscenely on top of leftover gravy. Now imagine it in your tummy, settling down gently on your stomach lining before being broken up by digestive juices and whisked away via your bloodstream . . . to block up your arteries or sit on your *hips*! Yuk.

Would you believe that we in Britain get an amazing 40 per cent of all our calories from *fat*? Yes, we eat the stuff voluntarily, as part of our daily menu! That 40 per cent consists of the 'hidden' fat in made-up meat products like pies and sausages, and the all-too obvious fat that clings to foods like chips, fried eggs, and takeaways. It also includes the fat in dairy products like cheese, full-cream milk and butter.

It is now widely accepted that the high incidence of heart disease in Britain is definitely linked to our appallingly high consumption of fat. So, it makes sense to cut fat for health reasons as well as to shed weight. However, it is not a good idea to try to cut out fat completely, as some diets suggest. Why? Because there are certain types of fat that are essential – even if only in small quantities – and some vitamins are present in fat (such as Vitamin D). It is also thought that polyunsaturated fats (in sunflower oil and oily fish such as herrings and mackerel) are good for your health. On the Fatfield Diet, these factors are taken into consideration.

But what about the taste of food? Does fat make it more palatable? For some people, heaven on earth is a greasy fry-up followed by a mug of milky coffee and a cream doughnut. If you are one of these, don't worry. Many of the original Fatfield slimmers thought that life would be grey and meaningless without greasy food. Honestly! Instead, they discovered that too much fat masks the real taste of chips, destroys the flavour of a cup of tea, and ruins the traditional British breakfast. Rather like giving up smoking, giving up eating so much fat gives your taste-buds a chance to savour food properly for the very first time.

SUGAR DOESN'T MAKE YOU SWEET

No, I am not going to give you another lecture on the subject of why sugar is bad for you. All I am going to say is that it contains absolutely nothing that does anything for your health or looks. There are no vitamins, minerals, fat or protein in sugar – just empty calories. About seventeen of them in every level teaspoon, a whole lot more hidden in foods like cakes, pudding, confectionary, many instant desserts, fizzy drinks and even canned vegetables.

Obviously, if you can cut back on sugar, you will cut back on calories. No, you will not go all weak and feeble if you stop having sugar in your tea because the body has ready supplies of glucose in the bloodstream and glycogen in the liver to spring into action when needed. No, it is not alright to replace ordinary, refined sugar with brown or demerara because they are just as fattening. If you are a honey fan, I am afraid that the bad news is that it is fattening too, although it has other properties which are beneficial.

On the Fatfield Diet, sugar is trimmed back as much as

possible. Which doesn't mean to say that you are not allowed to eat sweet foods. Fruits, puddings and some confectionary are permitted, but you must follow the diet-plans and recipes exactly.

PROTEIN: HOW MUCH DO WE NEED?

Protein, in meat, fish, eggs, cheese, and pulses such as beans, helps to build, maintain and repair the body. As I have already mentioned there was a time when high protein diets were extremely fashionable. Nowadays, scientists believe that we probably do not need as much protein as was previously thought – especially if we are adults who no longer need to 'build up' our bodies.

Indeed, some diet doctors advocate substituting complex carbohydrate meals (potatoes, rice, pasta – not sugar, which is pure carbohydrate) for the traditional meat or fish and two-vegetable meal.

This is certainly one way of saving calories. As I mentioned above, protein contains about 4 calories per gram, compared with 3.7 calories for carbohydrate. So if, for instance, you ate a jacket potato instead of a chicken leg with salad for lunch, you could save about 100 calories. If you normally ate the chicken leg with the skin on too, you would save even more.

However, while working with slimmers, I have found that eating some protein at each meal, in particular the first meal of the day, helps people to stick to a diet more easily. This is because protein definitely makes a meal more satisfying and prolongs that feeling of fullness. Protein foods 'burn' more slowly, sustaining energy levels for longer.

The problem is to find protein foods which are not bursting with fat as well. Cheese is definitely a dodgy one, since the protein it contains is mixed up with over half as much again in pure fat. Meats like pork and lamb are also dangerous for you can see the fat before your very eyes. Beef is possibly even 'naughtier', since the fat is often hidden in the flesh, giving just a slightly marbled effect to the meat. So, it is vital to look for very lean cuts and minced beef that contains only a small proportion of fat, and then to get rid of as much as possible during cooking. Even eggs are a problem as egg yolks are just about the fattiest thing you can eat apart from butter. In any case doctors now recommend cutting egg consumption to only four a week because of their high cholesterol content.

So which are the 'goodies' among the protein foods? They are fish, chicken (not the skin), low-fat yogurt, cottage cheese and pulses like baked beans, lentils and kidney beans. These foods are good sources of protein, so dishes containing them really do 'stick to your guts', and yet are low in fat, too.

On the Fatfield Diet, we have found ways of choosing and cooking other delicious protein foods to get rid of excess fat. We have also increased the protein power of cooked dishes by adding beans or yogurt. Many slimmers have slipped 'off the wagon' after having their nostrils assailed by the delicious smell of bacon sizzling away. That is one form of protein that you do not have to give up on the Fatfield Diet! Sounds good, doesn't it?

FIBRE: THE INCREDIBLE BULK

Do you want to feel full, instantly? Ignore those chocolate biscuits and crunch an apple instead. The reason apples are more satisfying than biscuits is because they contain fibre, so they take longer to chew. When each bit of apple reaches your tummy, the fibre absorbs water and you feel satisfied for ages instead of hungry again almost instantly.

So what is this magic stuff called fibre? It is the 'skeleton' or structural support that makes up all plants, from corn to cabbage. Although it does not contribute anything to our diet, it does help food pass through the body smoothly. A diet that is rich in fibre (in cereals, wholemeal bread, brown rice, wholemeal pasta, vegetables, fruits, bran) can help prevent diseases such as cancer of the bowel, diabetes, gall stones, diverticular disease and even heart disease.

In the West, we eat less fibre than people in Asia and Africa – around 20 grams a day compared with 50 grams. Scientists believe that we should try to increase our fibre intake to about 30 grams a day.

Fibre is incredibly useful stuff for slimmers . . . even if they do not like apples. Firstly, it helps make you feel full up without adding too many calories to your diet. That means you can sit down to a meal which includes a selection of fibre-rich vegetables (*not* boiled to death, which transforms the fibre into a mush) and get up from the table with a nicely satisfied tummy. Secondly, there is evidence that fibre 'chases' calories out of our bodies so they are not even absorbed. Although the number is small, around 5 per cent of the calories consumed, this is certainly a useful 'plus'.

The main disadvantages of adding too much extra fibre to your diet are the embarrassment of increased flatulence and the fact that it can prevent the absorption of minerals like iron and calcium. We must report that slimmers on the Fatfield Diet did *not* cause a sudden rush of wind through the Wear valley. Our diet is rich in fibre but not so rich that you will feel uncomfortable and lose all your friends as well as those much-needed minerals.

BIG IS BEAUTIFUL

If you use all the information above when you are planning everyday meals, you can in fact increase the size of those

31

meals while reducing the number of calories they contain.

That is what we have done on the Fatfield Diet. Here are some examples of menus that apply to Fatfield principles. Read them through before you turn to the next chapter for your Basic Diet Plan.

BREAKFASTS

Non-Diet Meal: 3 slices toast and butter with marmalade, coffee or tea, milk and sugar. Calories: 400

Fatfield Meal: 1 bowl bran flakes and a little skimmed milk, 1 slice toast with low-fat spread, 1 size 3 egg, 1 apple. Calories: 350

Non-Diet Meal: 1 fried egg, fried bacon rasher, fried pork sausage, 1 slice fried black pudding, 1 slice fried bread, 1 slice toast and butter. Calories: 1090

Fatfield Meal: 1 rasher grilled bacon, grilled tomatoes, poached egg, 1 grilled low-fat sausage, 1 slice grilled black pudding, 2 slices toast, low-fat spread, 1 pear. Calories: 550

LUNCHES

Non-Diet Meal: 1 round cheese and pickle sandwich with butter, 1 meat pasty, 1 can cola drink. Calories: 635

Fatfield Meal: 2 rounds wholemeal bread and salad sandwiches with 1oz (25g) chicken, 2oz (50g) tuna, 1 Diet Ski yogurt, 1 can diet cola. Calories: 410

Non-Diet Meal: 1 Big Mac and chips, 1 cup of coffee with milk and sugar. Calories: 840

Fatfield Meal: 6 chicken McNuggets, huge mixed salad, 1 slice of melon, 1 mug slimmer's soup. Calories: 345

SUPPERS

Non-Diet Meal: untrimmed grilled pork chop, chips, mushy peas, trifle. Calories: 1500

Fatfield Meal: trimmed grilled pork chop, jacket potato, broccoli, cabbage, cauliflower, green beans, slice of Toni's Amazing Trifle (*see* recipe, page 153). Calories: 550

Non-Diet Meal: Pâté and toast, scampi and chips, slice of Black Forest gâteau. Calories: 1400

Fatfield Meal: Clear soup, fillet steak and large mixed salad, jacket potato, lemon sorbet. Calories: 650

WHY YOU DON'T HAVE TO GIVE UP ALCOHOL

Any slimming counsellor will tell you that one of the quickest ways to lose weight is to give up alcohol. This is especially true for those men who normally drink a lot of beer. They only have to stop having 6 or 7 pints of lager or bitter every night to shed weight very rapidly indeed. They do not even have to stop eating fatty foods or sweets because alcohol is so high in calories that just cutting out one vice produces the required results, even if they carry on with their bad eating habits.

The sums speak for themselves: one half-pint of beer or lager contains about 100 calories (the same as a 'double' pub measure short drink, or a glass of wine). The increasingly popular strong lagers contain nearly *twice* that amount.

So, if a man is drinking 6 pints of beer a night, he is consuming at least 1200 extra calories, which is enough for a large meal. Over a week, that sum becomes a massive 8400 calories. With 3500 calories producing approximately 1lb of body weight, you can see that a chap can easily lose over 2lb a week by giving up drink.

The problem is that the vast majority of drinkers can only give it up for a short space of time, and then go back to drinking regularly. Result? The weight piles back on again.

On the Fatfield Diet I recommend drinkers to cut *back* on alcohol, but not to try and give it up altogether unless there are medical reasons for doing so. In my experience, it is more practical, and easier to cut down than give up. If you set yourself too many mountains to climb at any one time, you are much more likely to fail.

I must also say that, in my opinion, a certain amount of alcohol is *good* for you, particularly if it is in beer or wine rather than in spirits. The 'hard' stuff contains no vitamins or minerals, just 'empty' calories and it is all too easy to drink far too much of it, especially if you get into the habit of drinking spirits at home, where every tipple is a triple.

One of my favourite nutrition experts is the eminently sensible Dr Gaston Pawan, Senior Lecturer in Metabolism at the Middlesex Hospital Medical School in London. He has advised me for many years and has a refreshingly down-to-earth approach. Dr Pawan is one of the world's top authorities on alcohol and its effects on the human body. He believes, as I do, that drinking a modest amount socially is relaxing and helps to prevent stress, which is a major cause of heart attacks. He says, 'A couple of glasses of wine, or a pint of beer daily certainly won't hurt you. An occasional night out on the town with good company, a little good wine and lots of laughs is a far better tonic than anything your doctor can prescribe.' My own favourite drink is Guinness which I regard as a tonic as well as a delicious treat. It contains iron, Vitamin B and minerals, and contains about 100 calories in a half-pint measure. People often ask how I manage to stay slim and carry on drinking a pint of stout (sometimes more!) every day, but I simply make sure that I take the 200 calories into account on my Fatfield Maintenance plan. It is my treat, it does me good, and I make no apologies for enjoying every delicious sip!

CHAPTER FOUR

THE FATFIELD DIET: BASIC PLAN

The main principle behind the success of the Fatfield Diet is that slimmers *must* eat large, satisfying meals. Of our guinea-pigs from the village of Fatfield, the few who experienced difficulty sticking to the plan invariably had problems because they did not eat enough.

Remember: you will *not* lose weight any faster if you try to speed things up by eating less. You will only binge later on, making yourself feel guilty in the process. Don't do it!

Even if the amounts of food listed seem larger than you are used to, eat them up and enjoy them. I promise that you *will* become slimmer, healthier and feel wonderful.

The Fatfield Diet consists of a Basic Plan, plus ten variations of this plan:

The Basic Fatfield Diet Plan   This is suitable for men, or women, who lead a fairly sedentary life. That's people like me who combine looking after a family with a sitting down job, or those who do light factory work or run a home full-time. However, it is *not* suitable for men or women with more than 4 stone or less than 7lb to lose. They should go for the Steady Weight Loss or Quick Weight Loss diets in the next chapter. Also, men in heavy, manual jobs, should choose the Heavy-Duty diet in Chapter Five.

The Ten Variations   These cater for special needs and you will find them in the next chapter. They include plans for shift-workers, people who are in heavy, manual jobs, and vegetarians. In Fatfield, we found that the ten spin-off diets, together with the basic plan, provided a suitable diet for everyone. Where necessary, the plan was changed to cope with changing circumstances, such as a new job. Flexibility is vital while you slim. There is nothing wrong with switching plans mid-way. In fact, it can help give your metabolism a boost and prevent boredom, which is often the one thing that prevents slimming success. Never believe pundits who preach that you *must* stick rigidly to one diet, however limiting or boring it is – it just isn't true!

CONSULT YOUR DOCTOR BEFORE YOU START

No, this isn't the usual diet book 'cop-out' clause – it is sound common sense. These days, doctors are far more aware of the health problems associated with obesity and most surgeries now run some kind of preventive medicine plan such as regular health-screening sessions. So it is sensible to pop along to your doctor for a check-up before you try to lose weight. If you are very obese or are on medication for a specific problem, or are diabetic, it is absolutely essential to do so.

FREE VEGETABLE LIST: EAT AS MUCH AS YOU LIKE

There are certain vegetables which are so low in calories that you can eat them freely on the Fatfield Diet. Sounds like good news? Well, it certainly makes shopping a whole lot easier and it also helps you to enjoy the huge, hearty meals that are a vital part of the diet.

Why do we say this? Well, other diets sometimes tell you to measure out quantities of vegetables – 4oz (100g)

36

of cabbage or a solitary tomato. But since cabbage contains only 6 calories an ounce, and tomatoes contain about 12 calories each, you would have to eat a lot of either to put on an ounce. So, what is the point of limiting them? What's more, vegetables contain fibre which fills you up and is good for you.

Where possible, shop for tasty fresh vegetables. Nutritionally speaking, frozen are just as good but there is often a great difference in taste. Watch out for tinned vegetables, though, since they sometimes contain additives such as sugar or salt. If you want to save cash while you slim, check out local markets for cheaper vegetables. But always make sure that they look fresh, since valuable vitamins (particularly Vitamin C) can be lost if vegetables are left hanging around for days on a market stall. Greens should be *green* not yellow. Tomatoes, peppers and beans should be firm to the touch.

Serve vegetables very lightly boiled, steamed or as huge, satisfying salads. Use garlic (helps reduce cholesterol in the blood, so is a 'goodie' in itself), herbs, lemon juice or vinegar to make a dressing (*see* Fatfield Salad Dressing recipe on page 151). Do *not* add butter or oil in cooking. Honestly, you will never miss that huge knob of greasy butter on your cabbage, but your hips *will* miss it, with great results.

Here's your 'free' vegetable list:

Asparagus	Chicory
Beansprouts	Chinese Leaves
Broccoli	Chives
Brussel Sprouts	Courgettes
Cabbage	Cucumber
Cauliflower	Curly Kale
Celeriac	Endive
Celery	Fennel

Gherkins
Leeks
Lettuce
Mushrooms
Mustard and Cress
Peppers (red and green)
Radishes
Runner Beans
Shallots
Spinach
Spring Greens
Spring Onions (scallions)
Tomatoes (tinned or fresh)
Watercress

TEN WAYS TO SERVE THEM

Remember: the bigger the portion size, the better!

1. *Make sensational tomato sauce.* Simply poach chopped mushrooms and finely chopped onions in a saucepan of tinned tomatoes, with herbs, garlic and lemon juice. Serve with meat, fish or even on toast as a snack.

2. *Discover the delicious taste of raw spinach.* Use spinach leaves, washed and lightly torn up as the basis for a fabulous salad. Just toss them with sliced raw mushrooms, chopped celery, sprigs of cauliflower, lemon juice, vinegar and seasoning.

3. *Make cauliflower exciting.* Divide it into florets, boil very lightly and serve with a topping of tinned tomatoes which have been mashed lightly and heated through with herbs and lemon juice. You can do the same thing with leeks or braised celery.

4. *Check out the different tomato varieties.* Grill large beef tomatoes as a tasty, supersized accompaniment to meat;

enjoy the sweet taste of tiny cherry tomatoes on salads; and use the long-shaped Italian tomatoes in cooking. They are all delicious.

5. *Try braising*. Some vegetables taste delicious if baked in the oven in a little chicken stock. Try braising whole chicory, leeks or celery in a shallow casserole. There is no need to put butter on the vegetables. They will cook beautifully without. (*See* recipes, pages 149 and 150.)

6. *Make enormous salads* – and eat them at any time. You can have four or five salads a day if you like, as well as all your Fatfield Diet foods. Try cooked, cold runner beans with spring onions, radishes and chopped gherkins or cucumber and tomato with strips of red and green pepper. Or, you can serve up a hot salad – a mixture of cooked, leftover vegetables, whirled through the microwave and topped with Fatfield Salad Dressing (*see* recipe, page 151).

7. *Go Chinese with beansprouts*. Use this delicious, crunchy vegetable as a hot vegetable. Tinned beansprouts are in every supermarket and are just as low in calories (about 3 an ounce) as the fresh variety. You could even try growing your own. They are particularly delicious mixed with whole button mushrooms which have been poached in water mixed with lemon juice.

8. *Be an asparagus lover*. Just a few asparagus spears, cooked and chopped, add a luxury touch to salads. You can often pick up a bundle of asparagus cheaply in markets. They make a wonderful starter – eaten with your fingers and dipped into a little dish of Fatfield Salad Dressing.

9. *Try a Fatfield Stir-Fry*. You need absolutely no fat to make it since vegetables will sweat naturally. Just start by pouring half a tin of tomatoes into a non-stick pan. Chop

the rest of your vegetables and add to the pan gradually, cooking gently until just soft. Season to taste.

10.   *Be a vegetable artist*. Experiment with different ways of serving up salads and vegetables, to give a really colourful effect. Try piling individual heaps of washed, chopped, raw vegetables on a large platter. Or make a vegetable casserole, topped with sliced tomatoes, to accompany the Sunday roast. Don't forget – serve LOTS!

MILK: TRIM WITH SKIMMED

The Fatfield Diet allows $1/2$ pint skimmed milk daily for your tea and coffee. If you haven't tried skimmed milk before, you will find that it is much lighter, and thinner in taste, than the full-cream variety. It also has all the protein and calcium of ordinary milk. Most people find that they quickly begin to prefer it. It is certainly a taste that is well worth acquiring in terms of calories saved. Full-cream milk contains over double the calories (about 400 calories a pint, compared with 200 calories for skimmed).

BREAD: WHOLEMEAL IS BEST

Where possible, it is best to eat wholemeal bread on the Fatfield Diet. This is because, weight for weight, wholemeal is slightly lower in calories than white bread. It is also high in fibre, so a slice of wholemeal will make you feel fuller than a slice of white. But, you can also substitute brown or granary bread if you like, or one of the fibre-enriched whites. But where one slice of bread is given, this refers to a medium slice from a large cut loaf, not a thick chunk from an uncut one.

PORTION SIZES

When portion sizes are stated on the diet, you must stick to them carefully. Some foods, such as cheese and meat, are very calorie-intensive, so adding just a few ounces or grams more can jeopardise your slimming success. A pair of kitchen scales is a very useful investment, so you can measure portion sizes accurately. For convenience, in the diet plans 1oz equals 25g.

COOKING THE FATFIELD WAY

On the Fatfield Diet, we aim to cut right back on fat, so obviously cooking methods are vitally important. One of our star slimmers, housewife Rose Irwin used the diet as a great excuse to throw out all her old cooking pans and invest in a new set of non-stick ones: 'After having them for twenty years, it was time for a change,' she says. 'I had been using a couple of pounds of lard a week for roasting meat and potatoes, and now I don't use any at all which is good for our family's health as well as my figure.'

Here are ten tips for healthy cooking:

1. *Grill, don't fry.* From now on you're going to use your grill-pan instead of your frying pan. Make sure your pan has a grid, so meat can cook on top of the grid while any fat drips through the grid and can be disposed of afterwards.

2. *Skim off the fat.* When you're cooking casseroles, always skim off any fat before serving up the meal. If you prepare a casserole for supper the day before the meal, and store it in the refrigerator, it is very easy to whisk out any globules of fat using a slotted spoon before you re-heat it thoroughly in the microwave or oven.

3. *Buy lean mince.* It is not a good saving to buy cheaper, fatty minced beef. Instead, go for the leaner type, and pour off all the fat after browning it, before you add other ingredients. In a dish such as Fatfield

41

Shepherd's Pie (*see* page 139), we even advise putting the cooked mince on absorbent kitchen paper to blot off excess fat before combining it with beans and stock.

4. *Serve oven chips*. Yes, we really do allow chips on the Fatfield diet, but they are the oven kind *not* the deep fried kind. The calorie saving is considerable. Oven chips contain about 45 calories an ounce, compared with about 80 calories for medium, deep fried chips. The 'naughtiest' chips of all are crinkle-cut which have a high surface area which soaks up the oil, so the calories mount up to around 90 an ounce.

5. *Invest in a super set of kitchen knives*. You will need them for trimming fat off chops, removing the skin from chicken, and slicing vegetables. Where possible, buy meat from the butchery department of your supermarket instead of ready-packed. Then, you can ask the assistant to trim the meat *before* he weighs it, saving you extra pennies.

6. *Be an artful poacher*. Poaching – cooking food gently in water or stock – is an incredibly easy way of eliminating the need for added fat. For instance, mushrooms taste better and remain plumper if they are poached in water or a little chicken stock, and the calorie saving is enormous, about 60 calories an ounce. Or, try poaching an egg in a tin of tomatoes in a deep pan – you simply crack in the egg, taking care to keep it whole, and cook gently until both tomatoes and egg are cooked. Serve on a slice of toast for a quick and easy breakfast that only contains 200 calories.

7. *Never add butter or margarine to vegetables*. If you are frightened of protests from butter-loving members of your family, put the butter dish on the table so they can help themselves.

8. *Try grilling 'roast' potatoes and parsnips*. The traditional Sunday roast is definitely on the Fatfield menu. One easy way to save loads of calories is to parboil potatoes and parsnips, brush them lightly with a little melted low-fat cooking spread and place under the grill. Turn the vegetables a couple of times during cooking to crisp them up all over.

9. *Serve no-fat gravies and sauces*. Fatty sauces tend to smother the flavour of food, as well as adding calories. So, go for thin gravy made from a stock cube, tomato juice and water, or one of the sauce recipes on pages 151–2.

10. *Find creamy alternatives*. If you love cream in your cooking, there are lots of low-fat alternatives which you can choose instead. Try using low-fat natural yogurt (not the thick, Greek kind, which is higher in fat), or low-fat fromage frais.

CONVENIENCE COUNTS
No, you don't have to spend your whole day slaving over a hot stove to follow the Fatfield Diet. Convenience foods are recommended where they are suitable. Our Fatfield Team have tried and tested lots of different ready meals, packet soups, spreads and desserts, some aimed at slimmers, some not. Those they have found to be useful and delicious, are included in the diet.

EVERY PLAN IS MULTI-CHOICE
On most slimming diets the most limiting thing is the lack of choice. You are expected to eat a certain breakfast, lunch and supper on Day One, then another set menu on Day Two, and so on. On the Fatfield Diet, every variation gives a choice of breakfasts, lunches, suppers and treats, and it's up to you to pick the one you fancy.

This means that you get freedom and flexibility. You can go out and socialise, entertain friends, live a normal life. However, we do advise slimmers to vary their meal-choices as much as possible, so that they get their fair share of vitamins and minerals. Variety is the key to a healthy diet.

TREATS

You deserve a treat, so have one. Nearly every plan gives a list of treats to choose from. Make sure you don't go without these. Make 'treat-time' a bit special – when you're curled up with a book, watching television or just feel you need a boost.

TIMING

Eat meals when they fit into your lifestyle, bearing in mind that late-night suppers tend to stick around, on your hips! Don't leave long gaps between meals (fill them with 'free' vegetables, or a treat), and *do* make sure that you eat your breakfast meal as early as possible. If you simply can't eat it when you get up, pack it in a plastic container and take it to work with you so you can eat it during your first break. I do not belong to the school of slimming thought that advocates skipping the first meal of the day if you don't fancy eating it. You need a reasonable meal after eight hours of fasting to 'rev up' your body into top gear. If you miss it, you'll eat more of the wrong foods later on. Sorry!

BUY A FATFIELD PLATTER

To give your morale a pre-diet boost, buy yourself an extra large plate. A typical Fatfield Platter is oval, measures 18 inches (46cm) across and is designed to hold a *lot* of food. You may have something similar in your crockery cupboard which you are currently using as a vegetable plate. Amaze your family by using it for your own main meals. Pile on the 'free' vegetables and salads to make sure the plate is well filled up. Then sit back and watch their faces . . .

WHEN TO START YOUR DIET

When you have read through this book and studied all the diet plans, select the one most suited to your needs. At the weekend, shop for the foods you will need for the first few days of the diet, then start it on a Monday. Weigh in the same morning, and then on subsequent Mondays. Do *not* weigh yourself more frequently (and, even as I write this, I know that you will ignore me!) because you'll get impatient and frustrated. Expect to lose more the first week, less on following weeks. This is quite normal as the first few pounds that come off are fluid, not fat. Remember: the more slowly you lose it, the better chance you have of keeping it off.

SLIM WITH A PAL

Our Fatfield slimmers had the support and help of the whole group. If you can find someone to slim along with you, it really does make the going easier. Your 'Slim Pal' can be a partner, relative or close friend. If you would like to join our Slim Pals register, do write to the address given on page 108.

BASIC PLAN – RULES

EVERY DAY   You may have $^1/_2$ pint (275ml) skimmed milk for your tea and coffee, unlimited water, mineral water and diet soft drinks. Use an artificial sweetener such as Hermesetas. No sugar is allowed.

However, I would advise slimmers not to overload their system with too many fizzy drinks, diet or not. The very best drink is the still kind of mineral water which is truly delicious served with ice and lemon. Drink LOTS.

MEN   You should add 1 extra slice of wholemeal bread or a medium wholemeal roll with a little low-fat spread, 1 apple, orange or pear and 1 extra glass dry wine or $^1/_2$ pint beer or lager to your daily total.

FREE VEGETABLES   Choose them from the list on page 37. Eat plenty!

CALORIES   The diet contains about 1350 calories daily for women, 1600 for men. This may sound a lot compared with other diets, but you want the weight to stay off, don't you? It *works*, honestly.

BREAKFASTS (choose *one*, packed if necessary)

- $^1/_2$ grapefruit, with sweetener, 1oz (25g) bran cereal with a little extra milk, 1 slice wholemeal bread with 1 tbsp honey

- 1 slice wholemeal toast with small can (5oz/125g) baked beans, small banana

- 2 Weetabix biscuits with milk from allowance, 1 apple or pear, slice of wholemeal toast with scraping of low-fat spread

- 2oz (50g) unsweetened muesli with milk from allowance, topped with 1 chopped apple

- 1 size 3 egg on 1 slice wholemeal toast, grilled tomato, 1 orange

- Sandwich of 2 slices wholemeal bread with filling of salad and $^1/_2$oz (12g) Edam cheese

- Medium wholemeal roll with filling of 1 rasher of well-grilled streaky bacon or 2oz (50g) cottage cheese, 1 apple or pear

- 1 mug Batchelors Slim a Soup, 2 crispbreads with scraping of Marmite, tomatoes, 1 large banana, 1 carton Diet Ski yogurt

LUNCHES (choose *one*)

Sandwich made with 2 slices wholemeal bread or a medium sized wholemeal or granary roll with one of the following fillings and accompaniments:

- Salad (from 'free' list), $1/2$oz (12g) Edam cheese, Diet Ski yogurt and 1 orange

- Salad and $3^1/2$oz (88g) can tuna fish (canned in brine only, not oil), 1 small banana

- 1oz (25g) lean ham, 1 mug Batchelors Slim a Soup, large mixed salad from 'free' list, 1 apple

- 1oz (25g) chicken (no skin), large mixed salad, 4oz (100g) carton Shape Coleslaw Salad, 1 orange

OR
One meal from this list:

- 1 well-grilled beefburger in a wholemeal roll, large mixed salad, 1 small banana

- 2 slices wholemeal toast topped with small can (5oz/125g) baked beans and 1 size 3 poached egg, water-cress, mixed salad

- 6oz (150g) jacket potato topped with 4oz (100g) chopped cooked chicken mixed with 1 tbsp low-calorie salad cream, 1 apple

- 1 large slice of melon, 10oz (250g) chicken leg (no skin), grilled or roast, huge mixed salad or vegetables from 'free' list, 1 small wholemeal roll with a little low-fat spread

- 6oz (150g) any grilled or steamed white fish (e.g. cod, sole, plaice), with no fat added, 5oz (125g) jacket potato, 1oz (25g) scoop vanilla icecream with 10 grapes

Don't forget to pile on the 'free' vegetables and salad.

SUPPERS (choose *one*)

- 5oz (125g) lean pork chop or tenderloin, Fatfield Bubble and Squeak (*see* recipe, page 138)

- Steak and Kidney Casserole (*see* recipe, page 136), 8oz (200g) jacket potato, 1 apple

- Fatfield Shepherd's Pie (*see* recipe, page 139), 4oz (100g) peas, $\frac{1}{2}$ pint (275ml) custard (made up with skimmed milk and sweetener to taste added after cooking), and 1 small banana

- Pork Paprika (*see* recipe, page 137), 6oz (150g) jacket potato

- McCain Cheese and Tomato Deep 'n Delicious pizza, 1 apple and 1 pear

- Liver and Onion Gravy (*see* recipe, page 140), 6oz (150g) jacket potato, 2oz (50g) peas

- Bird's Eye Cod Steak in Wholemeal Crumb, 3 oz (75g) mashed potato, 3oz (75g) peas, 1oz (25g) scoop vanilla icecream, 1 small banana

- Piquant Mince with Dishy Dumplings (*see* recipe, page 140), 6oz (150g) jacket potato, 1 satsuma or small orange

- $^1/_2$ grapefruit with sweetener to taste, 3oz (75g) any lean roast meat, thin gravy, 3oz (75g) large chunks roast potatoes or parsnips, 4oz (100g) carrots, 3oz (75g) peas, Toni's Amazing Trifle (*see* recipe, page 153)
- 5 fl oz (125ml) chilled apple juice, Crunchy Wholewheat Lasagne (*see* recipe, page 144), 1 Diet Ski yogurt
- 6oz (150g) any white fish, grilled or steamed with a little low-fat spread (e.g. Gold Lowest) added, 10oz (250g) jacket potato, 1 apple or orange
- Indian Takeaway or Restaurant meal of Chicken Tandoori, plain boiled rice, onion rings, $^1/_2$ pint lager
- Chinese Takeaway or Restaurant meal of Chicken Chop Suey, plain boiled rice, 1 glass dry wine
- Steak House meal of lean fillet steak, jacket potato (no butter or soured cream), peas and 1 glass dry wine

Don't forget to pile on the 'free' vegetables and salad.

TREATS (choose *two* each day)

- 1 wholewheat crispbread topped with 1oz (25g) cottage cheese and scraping of Marmite
- 10 grapes
- 2 sticks celery with filling of 1oz (25g) low-fat cream cheese
- 1 apple or orange
- 1 medium digestive biscuit
- 1 mug Batchelor's Slim a Soup with 1 Ryvita crispbread

ALCOHOL ALLOWANCE

Every day, you are allowed $^1/_2$ glass dry wine *OR* $^1/_2$ pint beer or lager (if you are teetotal, you can have two 5 fl oz (125ml) glasses of unsweetened orange juice or tomato juice instead of these alcoholic drinks).

CHAPTER FIVE

YOU'VE NEVER EATEN SO MUCH!

Here are *ten* diets, based on the Fatfield principle of 'Eat More, Weigh Less' to cater for those slimmers with special needs. They range from a Vegetarian Plan, to an Anti-Bloating Plan created for women who suffer from fluid retention caused by menopausal or pre-menstrual problems. Men can choose from plans like the Boozers' Plan, the Heavy-Duty Plan and the Shift-Workers' Plan.

If you live alone you will love the Lazy Cook's Plan which offers a super selection of easy-to-cook dishes, and includes some of the excellent ready meals available from your local supermarket.

A CHANGE IS AS GOOD AS A FEAST!
If you wish to change your diet during your slim-in, do so. But first, make sure that the plan you are switching to is suitable for your lifestyle and starting weight.

Don't forget to vary your meal choices so you get a good variety of nutrients.

QUICK WEIGHT LOSS PLAN

This is *only* suitable for female slimmers who have half a stone, or less, to lose. It is perfect for women who want to shed weight rapidly for a holiday or special occasion. Stay on it for a maximum of two weeks, then go on the Basic Fatfield Plan for more steady weight loss. Portion sizes are particularly important on this diet plan, so do invest in some kitchen scales if you can. Don't forget to nibble away at your 'free' salads and vegetables between meals. The more you eat, the more likely you are to stick to the diet.

You can swap lunch meals with supper meals if you wish.

EVERY DAY $^1/_2$ pint (275ml) skimmed milk for your tea and coffee, unlimited water and mineral water. Use artificial sweeteners only.

MEN   Sorry, this diet is not for you.

FREE VEGETABLES   Choose them from the list on page 37. Eat plenty!

CALORIES   About 1000 calories daily.

BREAKFASTS (choose *one*, packed if necessary)
- 1 slice wholemeal toast with scraping of low-fat spread, 1 apple or pear
- 1 Diet Ski yogurt, any flavour, 1 large banana
- 1 size 3 egg, boiled or poached, 2 Ryvita crispbreads with scraping of low-fat spread
- 1oz (25g) any unsweetened cereal, milk from allowance, chopped apple on top
- small wholemeal roll with filling of 1 rasher well-grilled streaky bacon and grilled tomatoes
- 2 slices Nimble bread with filling of salad and 2oz (50g) cottage cheese

MID-MORNING SNACKS (choose *one*)

- 1 apple or pear
- 1 mug Batchelors Slim a Soup
- 1 Jaffa Cake

LUNCHES (choose *one*, again packed if you like)

Sandwich of 2 slices wholemeal bread with 'free' salad plus one of the following fillings and accompaniments:

- 1oz (25g) Edam cheese, 1 small banana
- 1 small jar of Shippams Beef or Fish Spread, 1 satsuma
- 2oz (50g) cottage cheese with chives and onion, a few grapes

OR

One meal from this list:

- Well-grilled beefburger in a bun (no onions) with 1 tsp relish, 1 orange
- Slimmers' Vegetable Broth (*see* recipe, page 145), 1 wholemeal roll with a little low-fat spread and 1 Kraft Cheese Triangle
- 1 mug Batchelors Slim a Soup, 3^1/$_2$oz (99g) tin tuna, canned in brine, 1 medium wholemeal roll with a little low-fat spread
- 1 slice wholemeal toast topped with small can (5oz/ 125g) baked beans, grilled tomatoes, 1 medium banana
- Citrus Salad in Yogurt Dressing (*see* recipe, page 131), 10oz (250g) chicken leg (no skin), 1 apple or orange
- 7oz (175g) jacket potato with one of these toppings: 3 tbsp baked beans, 1 carton Shape Coleslaw Salad, 1 carton Shape Cottage Cheese, 2oz (50g) cold, cooked chicken mixed with 1 tbsp low-calorie mayonnaise,

$3^1/_2$oz (99g) tuna in brine mashed with lemon juice and a little vinegar

SUPPERS (choose *one*)

- 3 fish fingers, grilled with grilled tomatoes, 3oz (75g) mashed potato, 1oz (25g) scoop vanilla icecream
- 3oz (75g) lean roast meat, thin gravy, 3oz (75g) chunks of roast potato, 1 Shape Fromage Frais or Shape yogurt
- 3oz (75g) lean boiled ham or gammon, 4oz (100g) tinned pease pudding, 3oz (75g) potato mashed with some of the cooking liquid, $^1/_4$ pint (150ml) Bird's Sugar Free Jelly, 1oz (25g) vanilla icecream
- Fatfield Bubble and Squeak (*see* recipe, page 138), 1 apple
- Fatfield Shepherd's Pie (*see* recipe, page 139). 1 satsuma
- 1 large slice melon, Spaghetti Carbonara (*see* recipe, page 135), 1 medium banana
- Liver with Onion Gravy (*see* recipe, page 140), 2oz (50g) potato mashed with a little skimmed milk
- Mixed grill: 1oz (25g) black pudding grilled, 1 well-grilled beefburger, 1 well-grilled low-fat sausage, grilled tomatoes

Pile on the 'free' vegetables!

STEADY WEIGHT LOSS PLAN

This plan gives an excellent weight-loss for women who have 3 stone, or more, to lose, and men who have just a small amount of weight to shed. In Fatfield, several couples followed this plan together. It is also suitable for teenagers who want to lose a bit of weight safely. Make sure you eat your treats. The alcohol allowance is, of course, optional!

EVERY DAY   You may have ¹/₂ pint (275ml) skimmed milk for your tea and coffee, unlimited water, mineral water and diet soft drinks. Use an artificial sweetener.

FREE VEGETABLES   Pile them on, choosing from the list on page 37.

CALORIES   About 1500 daily.

BREAKFASTS (choose *one*)
- 1oz (25g) any unsweetened cereal with milk extra to allowance, 1 slice wholemeal toast with 1 tsp jam or marmalade
- 5 fl oz (125ml) unsweetened fruit juice, 5oz (125g) can baked beans on 1 slice wholemeal toast
- 2 well-grilled rashers of streaky bacon, 1 slice wholemeal toast, 1 apple or pear
- ¹/₂ grapefruit with artificial sweetener to taste, 1 size 3 egg, poached or boiled, grilled tomatoes, 1 slice wholemeal toast with a little low-fat spread
- 2 Weetabix, milk from allowance, 1 slice wholemeal toast, 1 tsp jam or marmalade, 1 Diet Ski yogurt
- Sandwich of 2 slices wholemeal bread, Marmite and 2oz (50g) cottage cheese

LUNCHES (choose *one*)
Sandwich made with 2 slices wholemeal bread or a crispy roll with any of the following fillings and accompaniments:
- 1 jar Sutherland's fish paste, 1 orange
- 1oz (25g) Edam cheese, 1 dsp pickle, salad, tomato, 1 satsuma

- 1 well-grilled low-fat sausage, 1 tsp tomato ketchup, 1 mug Batchelors Slim a Soup, 1 apple
- 3$\frac{1}{2}$oz (99g) tuna, canned in brine, 1 tsp low-calorie seafood dressing, 1 apple
- 2oz (50g) cold chicken (no skin), diced and mixed with $\frac{1}{2}$ apple and 1 tbsp low-calorie salad cream, 1 Diet Ski yogurt
- 1 small carton cottage cheese with 1 ring chopped pineapple, 1 apple

OR

One meal from this list:

- 7oz (175g) can macaroni or ravioli, 1 slice toast, grilled tomatoes, 1 apple
- 2-egg omelette made in a non-stick pan with $\frac{1}{2}$oz (12g) low-fat cooking spread, 2oz (50g) lean ham, 1 mug Batchelors Slim a Soup
- Spaghetti Carbonara (*see* recipe, page 135)
- 10oz (250g) grilled chicken leg (no skin) with Barbecue Sauce (*see* recipe, page 152), 1 orange or apple
- 1 Beefburger in a bun (no onions), 1 small banana
- 1 10oz (250g) jacket potato, with topping of 2 tbsp baked beans or 3 tbsp cottage cheese, 1 apple or orange

Pile on the 'free' salads and vegetables.

SUPPERS (choose *one*)

- 3oz (75g) lean, cold roast meat, 7oz (175g) jacket potato, $\frac{1}{2}$oz (12g) knob low-fat spread, 1 frozen mousse
- Piquant Mince (*see* recipe, page 140), 4oz (100g) peas, 7oz (175g) potato mashed with some of the cooking liquid, 1 Shape yogurt

- 4 fish fingers, grilled, with grilled tomatoes, 7oz (175g) jacket potato, 4oz (100g) peas, 1 apple
- Fatfield Shepherd's Pie (*see* recipe, page 139), 4oz (100g) peas, $1/2$ pint custard (275ml) made with skimmed milk and artificial sweetener to taste, 1 small banana
- Aubergine Casserole (*see* recipe, page 142), 6oz (150g) jacket potato, 1oz (25g) vanilla icecream, 2 peach halves, canned in juice or water
- Greek Vegetable Soup (*see* recipe, page 132), 3oz (75g) any lean roast meat, thin gravy, 3oz (75g) roast potato, 3oz (75g) peas, 1 Diet Ski yogurt
- Bird's Eye Cod Steak in Wholemeal Crumbs, 3oz (75g) McCain oven chips, 1 apple or pear

Don't forget those 'free' vegetables.

OR *one* of these restaurant or takeaway meals:

- One portion Kentucky Fried Chicken with Coleslaw
- Chicken Tandoori with plain boiled rice
- Melon, 5oz (125g) fillet steak, 1 scoop vanilla icecream

TREATS (choose *two* each day)
- 1 slice wholemeal toast topped with Marmite or a little low-fat spread
- 1 fun size Mars or Snickers Bar
- 1 packet low-fat crisps
- 1 After Eight Mint and 1 small banana
- 1 mug of Batchelors Slim a Soup and 2 crispbreads with a little low-fat spread

ALCOHOL ALLOWANCE

You may have one glass of dry wine or $1/2$ pint beer or lager each day, or save it up for a night out. If you wish,

BEFORE

Russell and Vera Churnside look years younger now than they did when they started the Fatfield Diet. Since losing weight, Vera, 30, has taken a computer course (she passed with distinction), reached a very high level in aerobics and has studied dietetics. She is now our resident Fatfield Diet counsellor, running two Fatfield Slimming Pubs – at the Biddick Inn, Fatfield, and The Happy Wanderer, Framwellgate Moor. Russell, 32, lost 17lb. He recently tried hang-gliding for the first time. 'We both feel tons fitter,' says Vera, 'and our three young daughters are delighted with their new mum and dad.'

AFTER

BEFORE

AFTER

Erika Lowdon (*in the foreground, above*), lost 24lb on the Fatfield Diet and has maintained a weight of just over 9 stone for more than a year. She has taken up swimming and recently took part in a swimathon with her daughter Maureen and two grandchildren. She covered a distance of 1/4 mile – that's over 30 lengths of her local pool!

Erika, 63, underwent serious surgery during the Fatfield Diet experiment, and is certain that healthy eating helped her recovery. 'I feel strongly that everyone should try to improve their eating habits after a stay in hospital,' she says.

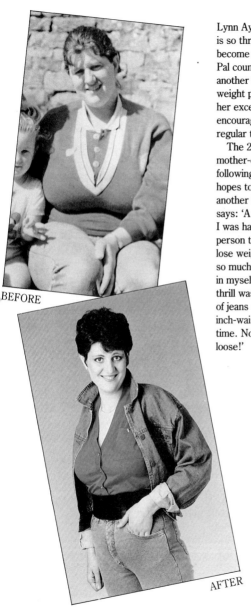

BEFORE

AFTER

Lynn Ayre lost 45lb, and is so thrilled that she has become a Fatfield Slim Pal counsellor – helping another mum with a big weight problem to shed her excess pounds, by encouraging her with regular telephone calls.

The 29-year-old mother-of-two is still following the diet, and hopes to lose at least another 2 stone. She says: 'A few months ago, I was hardly the ideal person to help someone lose weight. Now, I have so much more confidence in myself. My biggest thrill was to put on a pair of jeans with a size 32-inch-waist for the first time. Now, they are loose!'

David Jameson lost 5 stone on the Fatfield Diet. 'I was worried that I would miss out on things like big Sunday roasts, and drinks at the pub,' he says, 'but the diet lets you continue to enjoy your favourite treats and big hearty meals. That is why it works so well for men.'

A former athlete and sports teacher, David, 40, has now regained his lost form. 'When I was fat, I couldn't exercise,' he says. 'Now I play football, jog, and go circuit training.'

Marion Shergold, 46, started following the Fatfield Diet in March 1992 and she has now lost 4 stone. Her son, brave cancer victim Craig Shergold, couldn't be happier: 'I always wanted Mum to be slim,' he says, 'because she had high cholesterol and didn't feel very well . . .'

Marion's slim-in started after they were both filmed for a BBC-TV news programme during a fund-raising campaign for the famous Royal Marsden Hospital. Since losing weight, Marion's health has improved and she has recently written a book about Craig.

BEFORE

Brenda Taylor, 38, shed 31lb, and is still losing. She works shifts, but found that the diet can be easily adapted to fit in with the most awkward working hours. 'My daughter and husband love the recipes,' she says. 'I couldn't follow a diet where the meals weren't suitable for the whole family.'

Brenda is now able to wear much trendier clothes and has taken up horse-riding with her Fatfield neighbour, Vera Churnside. 'Six months ago I would never have dreamed of such an adventurous hobby,' she says. 'I am having so much fun now that I have lost weight.'

AFTER

BEFORE

AFTER

Susan Smith had so many food allergies that she feared that she wouldn't be able to follow a slimming diet. But we were able to tailor the basic Fatfield plan to suit her – and she has now lost 19lb.

Slimmers who have similar problems should show the Diet to their doctor or hospital dietician before starting.

Susan, 37, says: 'The diet has definitely helped reduce my asthma attacks. Anyone who has ever taken steroid drugs will know how depressing the extra weight-gain can make you feel. This plan really has worked wonders for me.'

Linda Philpott, 44, still keeps an old, size 18 skirt and the vast pair of shorts that she used to wear before she slimmed (*see picture on the back cover*). Now, she wouldn't be seen dead in anything unflattering.

Since losing nearly 3 stone on the Fatfield Diet, glamorous Linda has re-vamped her wardrobe to go with her size 10 figure.

'I'm so hooked on the Fatfield eating plan that I'm constantly experimenting with new ways of cooking the free vegetables you are allowed,' she says. 'The secret for me is never missing a meal. I'm sure that's why I have so much energy.'

you may substitute *one* of your daily treats for another ration of alcohol

ANTI-BLOATING PLAN

Just before a period, or during the menopause, many women experience unpleasant bloating. This is caused by hormonal activity in the body. It has been found that cutting back on refined carbohydrate foods (cakes, sugary cereals) and salty foods (bacon, canned soups, nuts, kippers) can help reduce this unpleasant symptom. Cutting down on cups of tea and coffee can also help. Certain foods, notably citrus fruits and cucumbers, can help 'chase' the water away.

This plan follows the Fatfield principles. It is marvellous for PMT sufferers and super for menopausal women. Several of our Fatfield slimmers switched to this plan for one week every month, just before their period.

EVERY DAY   You may have $1/2$ pint (275ml) skimmed milk for your tea, coffee and cereals. Limit cups of tea and coffee to 2 a day, and make sure coffee is decaffeinated. Other drink options include herb teas and mineral water (serve chilled, with a slice of lemon). Try to drink more water than normal, about 6 glasses daily.

FREE VEGETABLES   Choose them from the list on page 37, and be liberal with lemon juice when you are making salad dressings.

NB Use salt-free stock cubes to make gravy. Do not add salt in cooking. Instead, just put it on the table so the rest of your family can help themselves. You will find that the meals are tasty enough not to need the addition of salt.

CALORIES   About 1200 daily.

BREAKFASTS (choose *one*)

- $^1/_2$ grapefruit with a little artificial sweetener (leave it out if you possibly can), 1 size 3 boiled egg, 1 slice wholemeal toast

- 1oz (25g) unsweetened cereal, milk from allowance, 5 fl oz (125ml) unsweetened orange juice, 1 apple or pear

- 5 fl oz (125ml) unsweetened grapefruit juice, 1 carton natural yogurt with chopped apple and a few raisins

- 4oz (100g) reduced-sugar and salt baked beans on 1 slice wholemeal toast, grilled tomatoes

MID-MORNING

- 1 piece fresh fruit (choose from 1 apple, orange, pear or small banana, 1 large slice of melon or 2 plums), 1 Diet Ski yogurt

LUNCHES (choose *one*)

- 7oz (175g) jacket potato with $3^1/_2$oz (99g) tuna, canned in brine, lemon juice, 1 orange

- Sandwich of 2 slices wholemeal bread, lemon juice, 2oz (50g) chicken or turkey (no skin)

- 5 fl oz (125ml) unsweetened orange juice, 2 crispbreads with cucumber slices and 4oz (100g) cottage cheese, 1 apple

- 2-egg herb omelette cooked in a non-stick pan with $^1/_2$oz (12g) low-fat cooking spread, 1 Diet Ski yogurt

MID-AFTERNOON

- 1 Shape Fromage Frais, 2 crispbreads

SUPPERS (choose *one*)

- 3oz (75g) cold lean roast meat, 3oz (75g) mashed potato, made with milk from allowance, baked apple with filling of 2oz (50g) raisins, 1 crusty wholemeal roll.

- 5 fl oz (125ml) unsweetened orange juice, 6oz (150g) any white fish cooked in the oven in foil with lemon juice, sliced onion, sliced tomato, herbs, 7oz (175g) jacket potato

- 4oz (100g) grilled liver with sauce made from thin gravy and juice of 1 orange, watercress, 3oz (75g) boiled potatoes, 1 apple

- 4oz (100g) lean mince cooked 'dry', drained of fat and mixed with 1 small tin tomatoes, herbs and garlic to taste, 2oz (50g) (dry weight) pasta, 3oz (75g) raspberries with 1oz (25g) icecream

- 5oz (125g) lean lamb or pork chop, thin gravy, 3oz (75g) mashed potato, made with milk from allowance, a few grapes

- 3oz (75g) any lean roast meat, thin gravy, 2oz (50g) roast potatoes, 1 sliced orange with 2 chopped dates and a little lemon juice on top

- Fish Casserole (*see* recipe, page 137), salad from 'free' list with Fatfield Salad Dressing (*see* recipe, page 151), 1 orange

- 8oz chicken leg, skinned and casseroled in 1 can slimmers chicken or tomato soup, 1 crusty roll, a few grapes

ALCOHOL ALLOWANCE

You may have 1 glass dry wine or $^1/_2$ pint beer, lager or stout daily.

HEAVY-DUTY PLAN

This diet is suitable for men in heavy, outdoor work or fairly tough factory work indoors. It will help you slim down safely without feeling low or tired at work. The lunches can be packed or chosen from the canteen menu. If you prefer to go to the pub at lunchtime, there is a selection of meal choices for you. There is, of course, a daily alcohol allowance.

EVERY DAY   You may have ¹/₂ pint (275ml) skimmed milk for your tea and coffee, unlimited water, mineral water or diet soft drinks. Use sweeteners instead of sugar.

FREE VEGETABLES   Choose them from the list on page 37. Pile them up on your plate.

CALORIES   About 1800 daily.

BREAKFASTS (choose *one*)

- 5oz (125g) can baked beans, 1 size 3 egg, 1 slice toast
- ¹/₂ grapefruit, 1¹/₂oz (38g) any unsweetened cereal with milk from allowance, 1 slice wholemeal toast with scraping of marmalade
- 1 size 3 poached egg, 1 rasher well-grilled back bacon, grilled tomatoes, 1 slice wholemeal toast
- 1 well-grilled low-fat sausage in a small crusty roll with tomatoes
- 2 rashers well-grilled streaky bacon, grilled tomatoes, mushrooms poached in water, 1 slice wholemeal toast
- 2 Weetabix or 2 Shredded Wheat with milk from allowance, 1 apple, 1 small banana

LUNCHES (choose *one*)

Packed Lunches (don't forget to add plenty of salad from your 'free' vegetable list):

- 2 crusty wholemeal rolls with 2 grilled chipolata sausages, 1 dsp sweet pickle, 1 apple
- 1 medium Scotch egg, 1 small wholemeal roll, 1 satsuma
- 1 bap spread with mustard, 2oz (50g) lean ham, 1 packet low-fat crisps, 1 orange
- 2 slices wholemeal bread with one of these fillings and accompaniments:
  - 1oz (25g) lean ham, 1 Diet Ski yogurt
  - 1oz (25g) Edam cheese, 1 apple or orange
  - 2oz (50g) Shape Low-Fat soft cheese, chopped gherkins, 1 carton Shape Fromage Frais

Canteen lunches (ask for a large side salad *and* a big portion of green vegetables with your meal):

- 10oz (250g) grilled chicken leg, small portion apple crumble
- Lamb or beef hot pot, 1 low-calorie yogurt or a piece of fruit
- 4oz (100g) mixed cold meats, 10oz (250g) jacket potato

Pub lunches (please ignore the Shepherd's Pie, pasta dishes and curries on display – they are invariably fat and calorie loaded, sorry!):

- Ham or chicken salad, 3in (8cm) slice crusty French bread, 2oz (50g) hard cheese
- Small portion quiche, large mixed salad, 1 apple or orange
- Scampi-in-a-basket, 1 dsp seafood dressing, large mixed salad

SUPPERS (choose *one*)

- 3oz (75g) cold, lean roast meat, 7oz (175g) jacket potato, $^1/_2$oz (12g) low-fat spread, 1 frozen mousse

- Piquant Mince with Dishy Dumplings (*see* recipe, page 140), 4oz (100g) peas, 5oz (125g) potato mashed with milk from allowance, 1 apple

- Mixed grill: 4oz (100g) kidney, grilled tomatoes, 1 rasher grilled back bacon, 1oz (25g) grilled black pudding, 4oz (100g) mashed potato browned in $^1/_2$oz (12g) low-fat cooking spread, 2oz (50g) peas

- 4 grilled fish fingers, grilled tomatoes, 4oz (100g) McCain oven chips, 4oz (100g) peas, 1 apple

- Fatfield Shepherd's Pie (*see* recipe, page 139), 4oz (100g) peas, $^1/_2$ pint (275ml) custard made with skimmed milk and sweetener to taste, 1 small banana

- 4oz (100g) any lean roast meat, mini Yorkshire pudding made in non-stick tin, thin gravy, 3oz (75g) roast potato, 2oz (50g) peas, 1oz (25g) scoop icecream, $^1/_4$ pint (150ml) Bird's Sugar Free Jelly

- 5oz (125g) lean pork chop, Bubble and Squeak (*see* recipe, page 138)

- 1 small Bowyer's Cornishman's Pasty (5oz/125g), 4oz (100g) potato mashed with milk from allowance, 2oz (50g) peas

- Steak and Kidney Casserole (*see* recipe, page 136), 8oz (200g) jacket potato, 1 apple

OR

One of these Restaurant and Takeaway meals:

- 1 portion Kentucky Fried Chicken, coleslaw, barbecued beans, 1 apple or pear

- 6oz (150g) grilled rump or sirloin steak, fat removed, 8oz (200g) jacket potato, 2oz (50g) peas, 1oz (25g) scoop vanilla icecream
- Tandoori Chicken, plain boiled rice, 2 poppadums, 1 apple or pear
- Half a thin, medium pizza with vegetable and ham topping (NOT cheese!), huge mixed salad from salad table (avoid items with oily dressings), 1oz (25g) scoop vanilla icecream

TREATS (choose *two* each day)
- 1 fun size Mars or Snickers bar
- 2 digestive biscuits
- 1 crusty roll with a little low-fat spread
- 2 fingers of Kit Kat
- 1 packet low-fat crisps

ALCOHOL ALLOWANCE
You may have 2 glasses dry wine or 1 pint beer, lager or stout every day.

BOOZERS' PLAN

This diet will help most women, and all men to lose weight effectively. It allows some extra alcohol each day, which you can save up for one or two naughty nights out each week if you like. Sorry, it is *not* a drink-as-much-as-you-like diet! Try to make sure that you really enjoy the booze that you do have. If you are a lager drinker with a big thirst, it is always a good idea to have a refreshing low-calorie soft drink or glass of water before your first half-pint of booze, because the first drink just doesn't 'touch the sides' as it goes down.

EVERY DAY $^1/_2$ pint (275ml) skimmed milk for your tea and coffee, unlimited water and mineral water. Use artificial sweeteners only.

FREE VEGETABLES   Choose them from the list on page 37. Eat as much as you can.

CALORIES   About 1500 daily.

BREAKFASTS (choose *one*)

- 1 slice wholemeal toast topped with grilled tomatoes and $^1/_2$oz (12g) grated Edam cheese, 5 fl oz (125ml) unsweetened fruit juice
- $^1/_2$ grapefruit or slice of melon, $1^1/_2$oz (38g) unsweetened cereal with milk from allowance, 2 crispbreads with 1 tsp marmalade
- 2 rashers well-grilled streaky bacon, grilled tomatoes, mushrooms poached in water, 1 slice wholemeal toast with a little low-fat spread, 1 satsuma
- 1 size 3 egg, boiled, slice of wholemeal toast, 1 apple
- 1 Shape yogurt, 1 slice wholemeal bread topped with 1 tsp peanut butter, 1 pear
- Sandwich of 2 slices wholemeal bread, tomatoes, 1 well-grilled low-fat chipolata, chopped

LUNCHES (choose *one*)

- 1 medium bap spread with mild mustard, 1oz (25g) lean ham, salad with Fatfield Salad Dressing (*see* recipe, page 151), 1 large banana, Digestive biscuit
- Sandwich of 2 slices wholemeal bread, $1^1/_2$oz (38g) grated Edam cheese with 1 tsp tomato ketchup, 1 orange

- Crusty wholemeal roll with 2oz (50g) chopped cooked chicken, 1 packet low-fat crisps, a few grapes
- 1 McDonald's cheeseburger, 1 apple
- 1 pot Golden Wonder Pot Noodles
- 2 slices wholemeal toast with grilled tomatoes, 1 size 3 poached egg, 1 small banana
- 1 can Weight Watchers from Heinz slimmers' soup, 1 crusty roll, 3oz (75g) chicken breast with huge salad or vegetables from 'free' list
- 10oz (250g) jacket potato with one of the following toppings: 1oz (25g) diced lean ham or chicken, 2 heaped tbsp baked beans, 4oz (100g) cottage cheese with pineapple. Followed by 1 apple, pear or orange

Please pile on the 'free' vegetables.

SUPPERS (choose *one*)

Home-cooked meals

- Pork Paprika (*see* recipe, page 137) with 3oz (75g) potato mashed with milk from allowance, a few grapes
- Fatfield Shepherd's Pie (*see* recipe, page 139), 4oz (100g) peas, 4oz (100g) carrots, Shape Fromage Frais
- 4oz (100g) lean grilled lamb chop, thin gravy, 1 tsp mint sauce, 3oz (75g) boiled potato, 2oz (50g) sweetcorn, 1oz (25g) scoop vanilla icecream
- 6oz (150g) any white fish, grilled with lemon juice and sliced tomatoes, Leeks with Piquant Yogurt Sauce (*see* recipe, page 148), 1 crusty wholemeal roll with a little low-fat spread and $\frac{1}{2}$oz (12g) Edam cheese
- 3oz (75g) hot or cold roast meat, fat removed, 7oz (175g) jacket potato with small knob low-fat spread, 4oz (100g) peas, 1 frozen mousse

- 4oz (100g) (dry weight) pasta, boiled until cooked but still firm to the touch, tossed in mixture of 1 beaten egg and 2 tbsp fromage frais with 2oz (50g) grated Edam cheese on top, 1 apple
- 4 grilled fish fingers, 4oz (100g) oven chips, 4oz (100g) peas, 1 apple, 1 orange

Pub Choices
- Ham, chicken or tuna salad, no dressing, slice of French bread, no butter, 1 apple
- Small piece of quiche with salad or vegetables from 'free' list, no dressing, small helping icecream

Ready Meals and Takeaways
- Any Findus Lean Cuisine Meal with 8oz (200g) jacket potato and 1 apple or orange to follow
- Any Bird's Eye Menu Master Healthy Options meal, with 'free' salad and vegetables only
- 5in Deep Pan Pizza, with 1 large banana to follow
- 9 McDonald's Chicken McNuggets, with 1 apple or orange to follow
- Tandoori Chicken, with plain boiled rice and 1 apple or orange to follow

TREATS (choose *two* each day)
- 1 apple and 1 small banana
- 1 Diet Ski yogurt and 1 orange
- 1 crusty roll with salad filling
- 1oz (25g) Edam cheese and 1 crispbread

ALCOHOL ALLOWANCE
You may have 1 pint beer, lager or stout or 2 glasses dry wine or 2 short drink 'doubles' with a low-calorie mixer. But do try to have several drink-free nights each week.

LAZY COOKS' PLAN

This is a brilliant plan for men or women who want a diet with the minimum of fuss and bother. All you need to do is to stock up with meals from your local supermarket, and you are off! While you slim, you'll have loads of time for outside activities, so it is a good idea to join a gym or health club or practise the exercises in Chapter Eight.

EVERY DAY ¹/₂ pint (275ml) skimmed milk for your tea or coffee, unlimited water and mineral water, but go easy on the diet soft drinks. It is particularly vital to vary your meal choices on this diet, otherwise you will get stuck in a boring rut.

FREE VEGETABLES Choose them from the list on page 37. Frozen vegetables are just as nutritious as fresh, so don't feel guilty about using them to save time. But do buy fresh salads; it is so quick to wash them and serve them up to add bulk and taste to your meal.

MEN Add 2 extra slices wholemeal bread, and 1 8oz (200g) jacket potato or 3oz (75g) oven chips each day.

CALORIES About 1200 daily for women, 1500 for men.

BREAKFASTS

- Buy a Kellogg's Cereal Variety pack and have one pack every day with milk from your allowance, plus 5 fl oz (125ml) unsweetened fruit juice and 1 slice toast with a little low-fat spread

LUNCHES (choose *one*)

- 1 can Campbell's Main Course Soup, any flavour, 1 small crusty roll with a little low-fat spread
- Sandwich of 2 slices wholemeal bread with a little low-fat spread and 4oz (100g) cottage cheese
- 1 takeaway jacket potato with baked beans, cottage cheese or Mexican Bean filling, a few grapes
- 1 mug Batchelors Slim a Soup, 1 beefburger in a bun (no onions)
- Sandwich of 2 slices wholemeal bread with chopped hard-boiled egg and 1 tbsp low-calorie salad cream
- Any Boots Shapers pot meal with 1 large banana to follow
- 1 slice wholemeal toast topped with small can (6oz/150g) ravioli in tomato sauce, 1 satsuma

SUPPERS (choose *one*)

- 1 Ross Stir Fry meal, 1 slice bread with a little low-fat spread
- 1 McCain Deep 'n Delicious Pizza or 1 Findus French Bread Pizza, 1 apple or pear
- 1 large slice of melon, 1 Bird's Eye Menu Master Beef Curry with Rice or Chilli con Carne with Rice, Chambourcy Orange and Lemon Mousse
- 1 well-grilled beefburger, 3oz (75g) McCain Oven Chips, 2oz (50g) peas, 1 small chopped banana and apple, served as fruit salad topped with a few grapes
- 3oz (75g) lean roast meat, thin gravy, 2oz (50g) chunk roast potato, 2oz (50g) carrots, 1 Ross frozen mousse
- Any Findus Lean Cuisine ready meal with 3oz (75g) mashed potato made with skimmed milk from allowance

- Bird's Eye Menu Master Healthy Options Seafood Tagliatelli or Vegetable Lasagne, with 1 apple or orange to follow

Please do not forget your 'free' vegetables and salads.

TREATS AND ALCOHOL ALLOWANCE (choose *one* each day)
- 1 glass dry wine
- $1/2$ pint beer or lager
- 1 apple and $1/2$oz (12g) Edam cheese
- 1 Diet Ski yogurt with 2 Rich Tea finger biscuits
- 2oz (50g) vanilla icecream

VEGETARIAN PLAN

This is a delicious diet for men and women. Even if you are not a vegetarian, it is well worth trying out for the taste and novelty. You will find all the recipes in Chapter Ten which starts on page 131.

One or two of our Fatfield slimmers were vegetarians, and several were 'semi-veggies', who ate white meat and fish occasionally but no red meat at all. If you wish, you could swap any of the suppers given for a simple meal of a 10oz (250g) roast chicken leg, barbecue sauce, an 8oz (200g) jacket potato, some fruit and plenty of 'free' vegetables.

The diet is not suitable for Vegans, as it does include some dairy products.

EVERY DAY $1/2$ pint (275ml) skimmed milk for your tea and coffee, unlimited water and mineral water. Use artificial sweeteners only.

FREE VEGETABLES   These are obviously very useful for you, and I give one or two ideas on how you can use them imaginatively in the diet. Pile them on, not forgetting the Fatfield principle – eat more, weigh less!

MEN   You may have 2 extra slices of wholemeal bread each day, plus one extra 'treat'.

CALORIES   About 1200 for women, 1500 for men.

BREAKFASTS (choose *one*)

- 1oz (25g) any unsweetened cereal with milk from allowance, 1 slice wholemeal toast with 1 tsp marmalade, 1 small banana
- 2 slices wholemeal toast topped with grilled tomatoes and 1 size 3 poached egg.
- 1 Weetabix with milk from allowance, 1 slice wholemeal toast topped with 2 tbsp baked beans and grilled tomatoes
- Large bowl of fruit salad made by chopping 1 large banana, 1 apple, 1 pear, and topping with a few grapes and 1 small carton low-fat yogurt
- 1 Shredded Wheat topped with 1 chopped apple, a few raisins, and milk from allowance, 5 fl oz (125ml) unsweetened fruit juice

LUNCHES (choose *one*)

- 2 crusty wholemeal rolls, 4oz (100g) tub of Shape Pineapple Cottage Cheese
- Greek Vegetable Soup (*see* recipe, page 132), 1 crusty wholemeal roll with a little low-fat spread, 1oz (25g) Edam cheese, a few grapes
- 10oz (250g) jacket potato with Barbecue Sauce (*see* recipe, page 152) 2 crispbreads with a little low-fat spread and ¹/₂oz (12g) Edam cheese, 1 apple

- Sandwich of 2 slices wholemeal bread, mashed banana and 1 tbsp curd cheese
- Sandwich of 2 slices wholemeal bread, 1 tbsp baked beans, salad from 'free' list, and 1 packet low-fat crisps
- Citrus Salad in Yogurt Dressing (*see* recipe, page 131), 1 grilled Vegetable Burger (e.g. Dale Pak or Sainsbury's), 1oz (25g) vanilla icecream with 2 wafers
- 1 piece pitta bread, split and filled with 'free' salad and 4oz (100g) carton Shape coleslaw with 1oz (25g) chopped nuts

SUPPERS (choose *one*)

- Cauliflower cheese – have as much cauliflower as you like, with a sauce made from 1oz (25g) Edam cheese, 1 oz (25g) low-fat spread, 1 tbsp flour and $1/2$ pint (275ml) skimmed milk. Serve with grilled tomatoes, 2oz (50g) peas, 1 Diet Ski yogurt to follow
- Curry Creole (*see* recipe, page 143), 2oz (50g) (dry weight) rice, 1 apple
- Aubergine Casserole (*see* recipe, page 142), 5oz (125g) jacket potato, 1 medium banana
- 3oz (75g) (dry weight) wholewheat pasta with Fatfield Tomato Sauce (*see* recipe page 38), 1 crusty wholemeal roll, $1/2$oz (12g) grated low-fat cheese, fresh fruit salad of 1 apple, 1 pear, 1 satsuma and a few grapes
- 1 large slice of melon, Braised Leeks (*see* recipe, page 149), 2oz (50g) (dry weight) brown rice, 2 rings pineapple canned in juice
- St Michael Fresh Vegetable Canneloni or Casserole, 1 crispy roll
- 7oz (175g) jacket potato with topping of 1 5oz (125g) can baked beans, 4oz (100g) carton St Ivel Shape Garlic and Herb Coleslaw

- 4oz (100g) (dry weight) pasta, preferably wholewheat, boiled until cooked but still firm to the touch, tossed in mixture of 1 beaten egg and 2 tbsp fromage frais with 1oz (25g) grated Edam cheese on top, 1 apple

- Sharwood's Mild Vegetable Curry (14.2oz/405g pack), 1 frozen mousse

- 1 Vegetable Burger (e.g. Dale Pak or Sainsbury's), Fatfield Tomato Sauce (*see* page 38), 3oz (75g) oven chips, 4oz (100g) carrots, 1 large banana

TREATS AND ALCOHOL ALLOWANCE (choose *one* each day)

- 1 glass dry wine
- $1/2$ pint beer, lager or stout
- 1 Mars or Snickers fun size bar
- 2 After Eight Mints
- 1 crusty roll with salad from 'free' list

FOUR 'FREE' VEGETABLE IDEAS

As well as serving your 'free' vegetables cooked simply, or as salads, you can also dish them up like this:

1. *As a casserole* Peel and par-cook a selection of vegetables, pile into a casserole and top with tinned tomatoes, herbs, garlic. Cook in the oven until tender and serve with any of the meals above.

2. *As soup* Use a vegetable stock cube (or make your own) as a base, and add chopped, cooked or leftover vegetables. Purée to make a delicious soup to serve, garnished with watercress or parsley, before your meal. Eat as much as you like. Good vegetable combinations are:

leek, celery and watercress; carrot and tomato; cauliflower and cucumber.

3. *As crudités* Wash and slice a selection of vegetables and serve before your main course with a non-calorie dip of lemon juice, vinegar, crushed tinned tomatoes, garlic and herbs.

4. *As a stir-fry* Use a non-stick pan and cook through the watery vegetables first (sliced tomatoes, cucumber, beansprouts), gradually adding the others so you make a filling stir-fry without adding oil.

SHIFT-WORKERS' PLAN

When you work unusual hours, it can be very difficult indeed to stick to a low-calorie diet. You may be having your 'breakfast' at lunchtime and your 'lunch' in the middle of the night. Change-over days from one shift to another can leave you even more confused, perhaps eating two dinners in one day.

The one big rule to keep at the very forefront of your mind is that you need a good meal *before* you go to work, whether your job is in a hospital, factory, supermarket or office. This is because you need to make sure that you are at your best while you are working. You will therefore be less likely to reach for a snack when energy levels start to flag.

If possible do take packed snacks to work with you while you slim. Even if the canteen is good, you may still be tempted to eat the wrong things.

This version of the Fatfield Diet is deliberately very flexible. On rest days and weekends, you should follow a normal eating pattern with four meals daily. On working days, choose meals with the correct calorie values from the lists given. You are also allowed a 100-calorie treat every day, including alcohol.

EVERY DAY ¹/₂ pint (275ml) skimmed milk for your tea and coffee, unlimited water and mineral water. Use artificial sweeteners only.

FREE VEGETABLES Choose from the list on page 37. Pack LOTS of vegetables and salads in your 'goodies' box, together with your snacks, and take them to work.

MEN Add 2 slices wholemeal bread or 2 medium rolls, with a little low-fat spread daily, plus 2 extra Treats.

CALORIES About 1250 calories daily for women, 1650 for men (I would *not* advise shift-workers to try to slim on fewer calories than this).

REST DAYS AND WEEKENDS:
- Breakfast: 200 calorie meal
- Lunch: 300 calorie meal
- Dinner: 400 calorie meal
- Any time: 50 calorie snack and 100 calorie treat

NIGHT SHIFTS
First Night of Shift
- Breakfast (10–11am): 200 calorie meal
- Lunch (3–4pm): 300 calorie meal
- Dinner (about 1 hour before leaving for work): 400 calorie meal
- Supper (mid-shift): 200 calorie meal
- Snack (at home, before bed): 50 calorie snack
- Extra (any time): 100 calorie treat

Subsequent nights

- Breakfast (1pm): 100 calorie meal
- Lunch (4pm): 300 calorie meal
- Dinner (about 1 hour before leaving for work): 400 calorie meal
- Supper (mid-shift): 200 calorie meal
- Snack (at home, before bed): 50 calorie snack
- Extra (any time): 100 calorie treat

LATE SHIFTS

- Breakfast (10am): 200 calorie meal
- Lunch (12.30pm): 200 calorie meal
- Dinner (about 1 hour before leaving for work): 400 calorie meal
- Supper (mid-shift): 300 calorie meal
- Snack (at home, before bed): 50 calorie snack
- Extra (at any time): 100 calorie treat

EARLY SHIFTS

- Breakfast (just before setting off for work – or eat it at work, before you start): 200 calorie meal
- Lunch (mid-shift): 300 calorie meal
- After work: 100 calorie meal
- Dinner (with family): 400 calorie meal
- Supper: 50 calorie snack
- Extra (any time): 100 calorie treat

MEAL LISTS

200 Calorie Meals

- 1oz (25g) unsweetened cereal with milk from allowance, 1 large banana
- Sandwich of 2 small slices wholemeal bread, 2oz (50g) cottage cheese
- 1 size 3 boiled egg, 1 slice wholemeal toast

- 1 Diet Ski or Shape yogurt, any flavour, 1 apple, 2 crispbreads with a little Marmite
- 1 small wholemeal roll, 1 rasher well-grilled back bacon
- Large mixed salad from 'free' list with one of the following: $3^1/_2$oz (99g) tuna canned in brine, chopped apple, lemon juice; 8oz (200g) chicken joint, grilled or roast (skin removed); 3oz (75g) grilled ham steak; 3oz (75g) any lean meat
- 1 mug of Batchelors Slim a Soup, any flavour, medium crusty roll with one of the following: 1oz (25g) grated Edam cheese; 2oz (50g) chicken (no skin); 2oz (50g) lean ham

300 Calorie Meals

- Any Findus Lean Cuisine of 300 calories or less (calorie values are all marked on the package)
- 1 well-grilled low-fat sausage, thin gravy, 3oz (75g) mashed potato, 1 small (5oz/125g) can baked beans
- 4 fish fingers or 6oz (150g) any white fish, grilled, 4oz (100g) peas, 2 tbsp tomato ketchup, 1 crispbread
- 5oz (125g) lean lamb chump chop, grilled, 1 tbsp mint sauce, thin gravy, 4oz (100g) each broad beans and carrots, a few grapes
- Pork Paprika (*see* recipe, page 137), 1 apple or orange
- Fish Casserole (*see* recipe, page 137), 1 medium banana
- Fatfield Shepherd's Pie (*see* recipe, page 139)
- 5in Frozen Pizza, 8oz (200g) carton Eden Vale Vinaigrette Coleslaw, 1 crispbread
- 1 slice of wholemeal toast topped with one of the

following: 5oz (125g) can baked beans; 1 size 3 poached egg; 1oz (25g) Cheddar cheese; 2oz (50g) sardines canned in tomato sauce; followed by 1 apple and 1 pear or 1 large banana

Packed meals:

- Sandwich of 2 slices bread with salad from 'free' vegetable list and one of the following fillings: 1oz (25g) grated Cheddar cheese, 2oz (50g) (no skin) cold cooked chicken, 2 oz (50g) lean ham
- Crusty roll with filling of salad, plus any of the above sandwich fillings and 1 apple, orange, pear or small banana
- 1 mug Batchelors Slim a Soup, 8oz (200g) chicken leg (no skin), a few grapes

400 Calorie Meals

Choose any of the 300 calorie meals and add 1 slice bread or a small crusty roll with a little low-fat spread, or choose *one* of these recipe meals:

- 2oz (50g) any cooked, lean meat with Bubble and Squeak (*see* recipe, page 138)
- Piquant Mince with Dishy Dumplings (*see* recipe, page 140), 1 small wholemeal roll
- Bird's Eye Menu Master Seafood Lasagne or Chilli con Carne with Rice
- 1 portion Kentucky Fried Chicken, 1 portion Coleslaw, 1 portion Barbecue Beans
- Toni's Mackerel and Lemon Pâté (*see* recipe, page 132), 2 crispbreads, 4oz (100g) any roast meat (no skin), thin gravy

100 Calorie Meals and Treats

- 1oz (25g) any unsweetened cereal with milk from allowance
- 1 Diet Ski yogurt, any flavour, with 1 apple or pear
- 2oz (50g) any lean, cooked meat or small carton cottage cheese with 'free' salad or vegetables
- 1 small slice wholemeal toast topped with grilled tomatoes and $1/2$oz (12g) grated Edam cheese
- 1 fun size Mars or Snickers bar
- $1/2$ pint beer, lager or stout
- 1 glass dry wine
- 1 double pub-measure 'short' drink with low-calorie mixer

50 Calorie Snacks

- 1 sachet Ovaltine Options
- 1 mug Batchelors Slim a Soup and 2 sticks celery
- 3 large dessert plums
- Selection of chopped raw carrots and dip made from 1 small carton natural yogurt with mustard and lemon juice to taste
- 2 crispbreads with a little Marmite

Do not forget those 'free' vegetables and salads.

THE HIGH ENERGY PLAN

Sometimes Fatfield slimmers come to our groups feeling that they need to put some extra 'zest' into their lives. Perhaps they have been run down lately, or working so hard that they have neglected themselves. We recommend a two-week nutritional 'tonic' – the Fatfield High Energy Plan.

This eating programme is short-term, because it consists of six small meals a day instead of the usual three substantial ones with between-meals snacks. Most people find that they can organise their lives to accommodate this kind of eating for a couple of weeks, especially if it is going to give them noticeable benefits. The programme also needs a rather different approach to cooking – in fact, there isn't very much, as a lot of raw foods are served! However, you do need other kitchen skills such as chopping, using a blender, and even a juicer, if you have one.

On the plan you eat a lot of 'free' vegetables from the list on page 37, plus some other ingredients which might be unfamiliar to you including sunflower, pumpkin and sesame seeds and wheatgerm. Don't worry: these are easily obtained from the health food section in your local supermarket or department store. You will also eat more nuts, pasta and oily fish than on some of the other diet plans.

As a short-term programme, the diet is fun. The food is crunchy, munchy and full of bite-appeal. Each mouthful is a delicious eating experience.

You also get a chance to be creative: the salad dishes include unusual ingredients like the sunflower seeds mentioned above, fresh herbs and spices, and unusual fruits like mango and kiwi. Like every Fatfield eating plan, the diet allows you a *lot* of food. Each meal is satisfying – and there's always another one to look forward to!

The foods have been chosen to pack in the maximum nutritional power. They include vitamin- and fibre-rich wholemeal bread, fruits, fresh salads, pasta and nuts. Bananas are an important ingredient in the diet – they're packed with potassium. Lack of potassium is a very common problem in people who complain of feeling droopy all

79

the time. (Particularly at risk are those who take laxatives regularly, or high doses of aspirin.)

Meat and fish are served up too, but often as 'extras' on a salad or with vegetables, which are the main stars of the show. You *are* allowed some booze on the High Energy Plan. You can have half a pint of beer or stout (both good sources of Vitamin B), or a daily glass of dry wine. Sorry, but hard liquor is out because it drains energy and tends to make you more tired after the initial 'high'. The same goes for excessive coffee and tea as both are notoriously energy-sapping. Instead, drink more water or mineral water or even a herbal tea from the 'shopping list' below.

Switching to the Fatfield High Energy Plan from one of the other plans for a couple of weeks won't upset your weight-loss achievement. In fact, the change of 'pace' could help you shape up more quickly.

Don't forget that the key to well-being is a combination of diet and exercise, so do some extra brisk walking daily. Swimming is particularly beneficial if you are 'down'. We send our Fatfielders off to Aquarobics classes if they feel in the doldrums. A water workout really is a wonderful chance to let off steam, and does you tons of good. Try it!

WEEK ONE
EVERY DAY   ½ pt (275ml) skimmed milk for your tea and coffee. Drink lots of 'still' mineral water and the occasional cup of camomile or peppermint tea.

MEN   Add 4oz extra meat or fish (no fat in cooking).

FREE VEGETABLES   Choose them from the list on page 37. Don't forget to eat plenty!

CALORIES   About 1400 daily.

BREAKFASTS (choose *one*)

80

- High energy drink: 1 sliced banana, 1 small carton (5oz/125g) natural low-fat yogurt, 2 tbsp unsweetened orange juice whizzed up in a blender plus 2 crispbreads with a little honey for dunking

- 1oz (25g) unsweetened muesli topped with sliced kiwi fruit, chopped apple, milk from allowance, 1 small carton diet yogurt, any flavour

- 1 slice wholemeal toast, topped with grilled tomatoes, 2 tbsp cottage cheese, 1 dsp sunflower seeds, 1 pear

- 1 free-range egg, boiled or poached, 1 slice wholemeal toast, 2 satsumas

LIGHT MEALS (choose *three*)

- 1 medium glass freshly squeezed carrot or unsweetened pineapple juice, 1 apple, 1 small slice wholemeal bread with low-fat spread

- 1 large mixed salad (use unusual combinations of salad greens and raw vegetables) topped with one of the following, plus 1 wholemeal roll and 1 apple or orange:

  - 3oz (75g) tuna, canned in brine

  - 1oz (25g) toasted nuts

  - 3oz (75g) chopped chicken or lean ham

  - 1 chopped hard-boiled free-range egg
    (Dressing: use lemon juice, flavoured vinegar, herbs, black pepper but strictly no salt)

- 6oz (150g) any fish or shellfish, grilled or steamed, lemon juice, huge portion of vegetables, 5oz (125g) jacket potato topped with 2 tbsp natural yogurt

- 4oz (100g) lamb's liver cooked in a little olive oil with onions, huge portion of vegetables, 1 small slice wholemeal bread

- 1 mug homemade vegetable soup (use a mixture of vegetables in 1 large tin of chopped tomatoes, flavoured with herbs and garlic), 1oz (25g) grated low-fat cheddar cheese or 1 tsp chopped nuts, 1 crispbread

- 1 well-grilled beefburger or chicken leg (no skin), grilled tomatoes, large mixed salad, 1 small banana

- Sandwich of 2 slices wholemeal bread, 2oz (50g) chicken or lean ham, with lots of salad

SNACKS (choose *two*)

- 1 slice wholemeal toast with thin scraping of honey, cup of herbal tea

- 1 apple with 2 crispbreads spread with 1 tbsp low-fat cream cheese

- 1 large slice melon filled with frozen raspberries sprinkled with 1 tsp seeds, 1 tbsp natural yogurt

- 1 pear with 1 carton diet fromage frais

- 1 Harvest Crunch bar with a few grapes or 1 satsuma

- 2 crispbreads, 1 Delight Low Fat Dairy Slice, 1 small apple

- 1 small carton St Ivel Shape Cottage Cheese with Pineapple, 1 crispbread for dunking

ALCOHOL ALLOWANCE (choose *one*)

- ½ pt beer or lager
- 1 glass dry wine

WEEK TWO
EVERY DAY   ½ pt (275ml) skimmed milk for your tea and coffee, plus lots of mineral water.

MEN   As Week One

CALORIES   About 1200 daily.

BREAKFASTS (choose *one*)

- 1 medium banana, 1 small slice wholemeal toast with scraping of honey
- ½ grapefruit, 1 rasher well-grilled streaky bacon, grilled tomatoes, 2 tbsp sweetcorn, 2 crispbreads with a little low-fat spread
- 1 Shredded Wheat with milk from allowance, 1 sliced kiwi fruit, 1 small glass unsweetened orange juice

LIGHT MEALS (choose *two*)

Stir-fry of mixed vegetables with 1 dsp sesame seeds cooked in 1 tbsp olive oil with one of the following:

- 8oz (200g) grilled chicken leg (no skin)
- 6oz (150g) any grilled fish with 3oz (75g) boiled potatoes in their skins
- 3oz (75g) tuna, canned in brine

OR

Huge mixed salad topped with 1oz (25g) almonds, unsalted cashews or hazelnuts plus one of these:

- 2 tbsp cottage cheese or fromage frais
- 2oz (50g) tuna, canned in brine
- 2oz (50g) prawns or cockles

MAIN MEALS (choose *one*)

- 1 large slice melon, vegetable hotpot made from sliced mixed vegetables arranged in layers in an ovenproof casserole, topped with a layer of tomatoes, 1 small carton (5oz/125g) natural low-fat yogurt, ½oz (12g) grated low-fat cheese, cooked for 1 hour; serve with 1 small wholemeal roll
- 6oz (150g) any white fish cooked in foil with lemon juice, sliced onions and green peppers, 8oz (200g)

jacket potato, cauliflower, green beans, 2 tbsp carrots

- huge mixed salad topped with ½ avocado, sliced, lemon juice, 1 dsp sunflower seeds, 1 small wholemeal roll
- 5oz (125g) well-grilled lean sirloin steak, huge mixed salad with lemon juice dressing, 1 apple or orange
- 4oz (100g) roast or grilled chicken (no skin), broccoli, spinach, cauliflower, grilled tomatoes, 5oz (125g) jacket potato, huge mixed salad with lemon juice dressing

SNACKS (choose *two*)

- 1 pear
- 2 crispbreads with scraping of honey and 1 satsuma
- 1 mug homemade vegetable soup with 1 crispbread
- sticks of carrot, celery, green and red peppers with dip made from 3 tbsp natural yogurt, 1 tsp mustard, 2 tsp tomato purée, dash of Worcestershire sauce
- huge mixed salad topped with 2 heaped tbsp cottage cheese

ALCOHOL ALLOWANCE
As Week One

SHOPPING FOR VITALITY
Here's your diet checklist. Of course, you can also get most of these things from your supermarket.

Baker   wholemeal bread and rolls

Greengrocer   fresh fruit such as apples, pears, bananas, grapes, melon, kiwi fruit, mangoes; vegetables for salads and stir-fries – lettuce (look for cos, lamb's, radicchio, Chinese leaves as well as the ordinary round lettuce), watercress, red and white cabbage, carrots, radishes, turnips, sweet peppers, cauliflower, avocados, french beans, celery, mushrooms, potatoes

Grocer   free-range eggs, spring water, honey, herb teas, canned sweetcorn, tuna (canned in brine), natural yogurt, cottage cheese

Butcher   free-range poultry

Fishmonger   oily fish such as mackerel, trout; white fish – cod, coley, skate; shellfish – prawns, cockles, mussels

Health foods sunflower, pumpkin and sesame seeds, almonds, unsalted cashews and hazelnuts, herbal teas (such as camomile or peppermint)

THE PLATEAU DIET

Perhaps you've been slimming successfully for some time, but still have some weight left which just refuses to budge.

During our Fatfield slim-in for the BBC 'Bazaar' programme, a few of our slimmers did get stuck on a dieting 'plateau'. They had lost weight slowly but surely (the best way!) for several months, but suddenly found that no weight-loss registered at our weekly weigh-ins.

So, I devised this special diet to help rev up their sluggish metabolism and encourage their bodies to start 'burning' calories again.

Week One is a maintenance plan of 1500 calories designed to give the body a 'holiday' from dieting. It is divided up into four meals instead of three, to liven up your system. Walk briskly for one hour each day, too.

Week Two allows 1200 calories. Exercise this week should include a gentle aerobic activity such as swimming three times a week.

Repeat the two Weeks alternately until the weight

starts moving again, then choose one of the other diets in this book.

WEEK ONE

EVERY DAY　You can have ½ pt (275ml) skimmed milk for your tea and coffee and unlimited water and mineral water. Use artificial sweeteners only.

MEN　(and women with more than 3 stone (19kg) to lose). You can have 2 extra slices of wholemeal bread daily with a little low-fat spread.

FREE VEGETABLES　Choose from the list on page 37. Eat as much as you can.

CALORIES　About 1500 daily for women, 1700 for men and women with more than 3 stone (19kg) to lose.

NOW CHOOSE　Each day choose *one* Breakfast, *two* Light Meals, *one* Main Meal and *one* Treat. Eat them whenever you like.

BREAKFASTS (choose *one*)

- 1 poached egg, grilled tomatoes, 1 slice of wholemeal toast, watercress and cucumber
- ½ grapefruit or 1 slice of melon, 1oz (25g) unsweetened cereal with milk from allowance, 2 crispbreads with 1 tsp marmalade
- 2 slices of wholemeal toast topped with grilled tomatoes and 1 rasher grilled streaky bacon, watercress or cucumber slices
- 1 slice of wholemeal toast topped with 1 small can (5oz/125g) baked beans, grilled tomatoes

LIGHT MEALS (choose *two*)
Don't forget to add huge mixed salads and vegetables from the 'free' list on page 37.

- Greek Vegetable Soup (*see* recipe, page 132), 1 wholemeal roll, 1 small banana

- Any Findus Lean Cuisine meal, plus 1 apple, pear or orange

- Citrus Salad in Lemon Dressing, 1 slice wholemeal bread, 1 satsuma or clementine

- *Sandwiches* Allow 2 slices of wholemeal bread with filling of salad from the 'free' list (page 37) and one of these accompaniments:

  - 2oz (50g) lean ham or chicken (no skin) with 1 tsp sweet pickle

  - 4oz (100g) cottage cheese with chives

  - 1 large mashed banana with a sprinkling of cinnamon

  - 3 orange slices and 1 tbsp Shape Soft Cheese. Add 1 can (10.4oz/295g) Weight Watchers from Heinz soup

- *Baked potatoes* Allow one 10oz (250g) potato, scrubbed and baked, with one of these toppings:

  - 1 small carton (5oz/125g) natural, low-fat yogurt with sprinkling of curry powder and lemon juice

  - 2 tbsp baked beans, sliced tomatoes

  - 1 small carton (5oz/125g) Shape coleslaw salad

  - 1 small can tomatoes (8oz/227g) with 2oz (50g) chopped prawns or shrimps

- *Cold platter* Salad from 'free' list (page 37) with sliced hard-boiled egg, 2 tbsp sweetcorn **or** 1 small carton (4oz/100g) cottage cheese with chives or pineapple, onion rings, orange slices, 2 tbsp raisins

MAIN MEALS (choose *one*)
Don't forget your 'free' vegetables and salads (page 37)

Home Cooked

- 3oz (75g) lean roast meat, 3oz (75g) dry roast potatoes cooked the Fatfield way (see page 43), Toni's Amazing Trifle (*see* recipe, page 153)

- 6oz (150g) any white fish, grilled with lemon juice and sliced tomatoes, 8oz (200g) baked potato, 1 baked apple with 2 tbsp fromage frais

- 1 well-grilled beefburger or vegeburger, 3oz (75g) oven chips, 1 small can (7.6oz/215g) spaghetti in tomato sauce, 1 scoop vanilla icecream

Ready Meals and Takeaways

- Any Findus Lean Cuisine or Weight Watchers from Heinz meal with 8oz (200g) baked potato and 1 apple or orange to follow

- Bird's Eye Menu Master Chicken Casserole or Chinese Chicken and Rice, 2 tbsp carrots, 1 small wholemeal roll

- St Michael Potato and Bacon Gratin or Mushroom and Pasta Bake, 2 tbsp peas, 1½oz (35g) vanilla icecream

- Tandoori Chicken or Chicken Tikka, 3 tbsp plain boiled rice, 1 small banana

- Haddock in Batter from chippie, with unlimited salad and vegetables only

- Prawn Chop Suey, 2 tbsp plain boiled rice, 1 apple

Restaurants

- ½ melon with ginger, 3oz (75g) any cold lean meat, 10oz (250g) jacket potato topped with 2 tbsp baked beans, 1 apple or orange

- 6oz (175g) fillet or rump steak, 1 small baked potato with no topping

- Melon cocktail, roast chicken and unlimited 'free' vegetables

TREATS (choose *one*)

- 1 glass of dry wine
- 2 'short' drinks (pub measure) with low-calorie mixers only
- ½pt (275ml) beer or lager (not strong lager)
- 1 fun size Mars or Snickers bar
- 1 small digestive biscuit

WEEK TWO
EVERY DAY   ½ pt (275ml) skimmed milk for your tea and coffee, unlimited water and mineral water. Use artificial sweeteners only.

FREE VEGETABLES   Choose from the list on page 37. Eat as much as you can.

MEN   (and women with more than 3 stone (19kg) to lose). Add 2 slices of wholemeal bread, ½ pt (275ml) beer or lager or 1 glass wine

NOW CHOOSE   Each day choose *one* Breakfast, *one* Light Meal, *one* Main Meal and *one* Treat

BREAKFASTS (choose *one*)

- 1 small glass unsweetened orange juice, 1 slice of wholemeal toast with Marmite, 1 apple
- 1 small wholemeal roll with 1 rasher grilled back bacon and grilled tomatoes
- 1 small carton (5oz/125g) natural low-fat yogurt whizzed in the blender with 1 tbsp wheatgerm, 1 large chopped banana

- 2 crispbreads, grilled tomatoes, 2oz (50g) mushrooms poached in water, 1 poached egg, watercress
- ½ grapefruit, grilled with a pinch of cinnamon on top, 1 slice of wholemeal toast with 1 tsp honey, 1 low-calorie fruit yogurt, any flavour

LIGHT MEALS (choose *one*)
Sandwich meals
Use 2 slices of wholemeal bread or 2 small crispy rolls with salad and one of these fillings:

- 2 sardines, drained and mashed with lemon juice, 1 tbsp natural low-fat yogurt, diced cucumber, red and green peppers
- 1 pear, cored and sliced, lemon juice, 1oz (25g) chopped lean ham
- 1oz (25g) grated Edam with 1 tsp sweet pickle
  Add: 1 apple, orange, pear or small banana

Soup meals
- Any Heinz Whole Soup or Farmhouse Soup with 1 small wholemeal roll
- Any Weight Watchers from Heinz soup with 1 small wholemeal roll and 1 carton low-calorie fruit yogurt, any flavour
- Greek Vegetable Soup (*see* recipe, page 132) with 1 slice wholemeal bread, 1 banana, 1 satsuma or clementine

Baked potato meals
Cook one 10oz (275g) baked potato, and top with one of the following (don't forget that 'free' salad):

- 2 tbsp natural low-fat yogurt and ½oz (12g) grated Edam cheese

- 2 tbsp baked beans and chopped tomato
- 4 tbsp cottage cheese with chives or pineapple

MAIN MEALS (choose *one*)

- Liver and Onion Gravy (*see* recipe, page 140), 3oz (75g) potato, mashed with skimmed milk from allowance
- 3oz (75g) any cooked, lean meat or 5oz (125g) any grilled white fish with 3oz (75g) potato mashed with skimmed milk from allowance, 2 tbsp peas, thin gravy (for meat only, make it with a stock cube), with a frozen mousse or fromage frais to follow
- Any Findus Lean Cuisine or Weight Watchers from Heinz meal with 2 pieces of fresh fruit (apple, orange, pear, small banana, 2 plums or a large slice of melon) to follow
- Curry Creole (*see* recipe, page 143), 3 tbsp boiled rice
- 1 well-grilled beefburger, grilled tomatoes, Fatfield Bubble and Squeak (*see* recipe, page 138)
- 1 large slice of melon, Bird's Eye Cod Steak in Butter, mushroom or parsley sauce, 10oz (250g) jacket potato, 1 apple or orange

Try to avoid eating out this week. If you must, go to a carvery and have chicken or turkey, 'free' vegetables and a fruit sorbet or fresh fruit to follow.

TREATS (choose *one*)

- ½ pt (275ml) beer or lager **or** 1 glass of dry wine
- 2 'short' drinks (pub measure) with low-calorie mixers
- 1 fun size Mars or Snickers bar
- 1 individual meringue nest topped with ½ tbsp low-fat fromage frais and 2oz (50g) strawberries or raspberries

CHAPTER SIX

HOW OUR SLIMMERS COPED

Here are some inspiring stories from our original group of Fatfield Slimmers. Anyone who has ever been overweight will recognise many of the problems that these super people had before they changed their eating habits. In some cases, the pounds had piled on gradually over the years. In others, there were medical or emotional reasons why they had put on weight.

As the pounds dropped off, it was exciting to see how much healthier and more active everyone became. Toni, my assistant, and I noticed that people seemed busier and busier. People who had been coming along to our regular weigh-ins wearing ordinary clothes, suddenly started turning up in skin-tight leotards and cycling shorts! Not only that, they had fitted in an aquafit or exercise session before our meeting.

The social scene in Fatfield is pretty active anyway, but we found that some slimmers had so much energy they were able to dance the night away, even after a tough day at work.

Vera Churnside joined a car maintenance class and braved an army assault course along with Linda Philpott and a group of fellow Fatfield slimmers. Which all proves that the right diet makes you *feel* terrific as well as *look* tons better!

Name: **David Jameson**
Age: 40   *Occupation*: Sales Representative
Height: 6ft 2in
Starting weight: 17st 7lb   *Weight after 24 weeks*: 13st 7lb

September 19 1991 was Dave Jameson's thirty-ninth birthday. That morning, as he heaved his huge 17½ stone bulk onto his bathroom scales, he decided that he had just twelve months to change his life, and his fitness level:

'I reckoned that I could either be fat and forty, or fit and forty,' says Dave, from Washington, Tyne and Wear. 'But, after checking my weight on those scales and looking in the mirror, the former seemed the most likely!'

Since being made redundant from his job six months earlier, Dave had become a 'couch potato', watching television most of the day and spending the evenings munching his way through chips and takeaways.

'Noone would have believed that I was a former PE teacher with a string of sporting records and qualifications to my name,' he says. 'I was nothing but a big fat lump.' For someone who was once the English Schools junior mile champ, represented Durham and Loughborough College at rugby and was a county basketball star, it was depressing to say the least. He was also demoralised after those long months without work.

Dave's wife Julie had joined our Fatfield group, and Dave decided that he would give himself a birthday present and come along too.

'I gave myself six months to see some improvement,' he says. Within three weeks his weight was down to 16st 2lb, and he had started swimming and weight-training sessions at the local leisure centre.

We started Dave off on the Heavy-Duty diet. He needed plenty of the right kind of food because he is so tall and was determined to take plenty of exercise as he slimmed. 'I found that I was actually eating more than before,' he says, 'but I was concerned that the diet might cost more as we were obviously strapped for cash.'

He needn't have worried; the diet is less expensive than he thought, and there is no waste as every meal is a huge one.

'As the weight dropped off, I increased my exercise level,' says Dave. 'I started jogging three times a week, and took up football and squash. I quickly began to feel a whole lot better about myself, even though I still couldn't find work.'

He reached his goal after six months. His weight has gone up slightly since then as he has increased his fitness routine to six or seven sessions of either super circuit training, squash, jogging or swimming every week. This means that his body has altered considerably, with more muscle and less fat, but a much leaner shape.

Recently, Dave landed a great job and is now back in full-time employment. 'I make sure that I don't spend too much time sitting in the car,' he says. 'I drive to a central point, and walk or jog to appointments and I play football every Saturday for a local team.' Last season, he scored 20 goals. Some couch potato!

Name: **Julie Robson**
Age: 29   *Occupation*: Housewife   *Height*: 5ft 3in
Starting weight: 14st 8lb   *Weight now*: 9st 9lb

Pretty Julie Robson is pictured on the front cover of this new edition of *The Fatfield Diet*. She looks slim, happy and full of confidence.

Yet when she started the Fatfield Diet in February 1991, Julie was very overweight, depressed and eating all the wrong foods.

'My weight had become a kind of shield to hide behind,' she says. 'My husband, Jimmy, was killed in a car crash in December 1989, and ever since I had just neglected myself. I cooked three good meals for my daughter Stephanie but never sat down to eat with her. Instead, I just forgot about eating until I was really hungry, and then stuffed myself with leftovers and snacks.'

Her grief was so intense that she spent most evenings crying in front of the TV, with a pile of sandwiches or biscuits on her lap. 'I used the food to deaden the pain,' she says. 'I didn't care what I looked like, so getting fat never worried me.'

It wasn't until her clothes became unbearably tight that Julie finally realised that she would have to do something drastic. She joined our Fatfield group which meets every Wednesday at the Biddick Inn in the village. Successful Fatfield slimmer Vera Churnside is the group's counsellor.

'My sister Sheila was already a member, so I knew the club was fun, but I didn't think the diet would do much for me,' she says.

When she weighed in after the very first week, she found she had lost 8lb. Over the coming weeks, she felt a lot healthier, happier and ready to mix more. Vera noticed that even her body language altered: 'Instead of sitting hunched up over a diet soft drink, Julie looked alert and confident,' she says. 'Her posture improved and she started to laugh more.'

'The foods are so delicious on the diet that I actually started to look forward to meals,' says Julie. 'I sat down at the table and ate them with Stephanie, and took a pride in the way I served them up. Food became fun again.'

She lost weight steadily at the rate of around 2lb a week and reached her goal in October 1992.

Despite her new size 12 figure, shy Julie was reluctant

to buy some new clothes: 'I felt it would be disloyal to Jimmy to start getting all dolled up again,' she says. 'But then I came to London to be photographed, and felt that it was time to change.

'I have realised that I can learn to live with my grief and still be a caring mum and have some social life. The diet has given me strength to cope, as well as helped me slim. I think Jimmy would be proud of me.'

Name: **Marion Shergold**
Age: 46 *Occupation*: Housewife and Author
Height: 5ft 2½in
Starting weight: **15st 8lb** *Weight after 1 year*: **11st 6lb**

Brave Marion Shergold from Carshalton, Surrey, neglected her own needs when her son Craig nearly died from a brain tumour. Craig, thirteen, captured the imagination of the world when he collected more than 50 million get-well cards, a record.

Naturally, Marion's first priority was to care for her son during his long illness. So, from February 1989 onwards, she spent seventeen months by his bedside at the famous Royal Marsden Hospital in London. Instead of eating proper meals, she grabbed snacks and takeaways when there was time. Not surprisingly, she often suffered from indigestion, and her diet was fat-loaded and lacking in vitamins and minerals.

'My husband Ernie and I organised our visits in shifts,' she says. 'When Ernie finished work he would take over from me, bringing some fish and chips or a Chinese meal. I never cared what I ate, and I lived in comfortable track-suits wich expanded to fit my ever-increasing waistline!' Over the three long years that Craig was seriously ill, Marion's weight gradually crept up from 10½ stone to over 15½ stone.

'Luckily, Craig had a life-saving operation in America and I was, at last, able to look at my own health problems. My doctor was horrified with my weight-gain. Stress had pushed up my cholesterol to a dangerously high level and I had asthma attacks.'

I put Marion on the Fatfield Diet in March 1992, and she has never looked back. By last summer, she had lost 2 stone and she is now heading down towards her goal of 10 stone.

'It was a revelation,' she says. 'I love the occasional whisky, and I can have quite a few on the diet! I have cereal or egg and bacon for breakfast, a salad or sandwich lunch and a filling supper. The diet fits in well with our lifestyle. Ernie has lost 1½ stone without even trying, and Craig has lost 6lb. This is excellent as he has spent so many months lying down and sitting around that he has been unable to get the kind of exercise a boy of his age needs.

'My doctor is delighted because my cholesterol level is now normal, and my asthma never troubles me.'

Last September, Craig started back at school, so Marion was able to go out more. She now goes to a fitness centre for exercise sessions, and has just spent a week at Henlow Grange health farm. Noone deserved that week more!

She has also written a book about her experiences: 'A year ago, I felt too tired and low to do anything except care for Craig. Now, I have actually managed to write the full story of Craig's exceptional courage. It comes out in November 1993, and I am determined to be a slim 10 stone for the launch party.'

Marion is a marvellous lady who has had to cope with more than her fair share of troubles, so I'm sure losing that extra 21lb won't be a problem!

Name: **Linda Philpott**
Age: 44   *Occupation*: Supermarket Department Instructor
Height: 5ft 3in
Starting weight: **11st 6lb**   *Weight after 20 weeks*: **9st 7lb**

It's hard to believe that glamorous Linda has three daughters and two small grandchildren. She is slim, stunningly attractive and looks about thirty. Despite holding down a full-time job, she manages to fit in swimming, aerobics, stepping classes and circuit training! Her wardrobe is full of lovely tight-fitting Lycra dresses, shorts and leotards. There isn't an ounce of spare flesh on her beautifully toned-up body.

It's hard to believe that when she had her daughter Paula, who's now twenty-six , Linda thought she would never be slim gain: 'I expanded to 12 stone and just couldn't slim down,' she says. 'So, when Vicky came along four years later, I was determined to shape up.'

However, things didn't turn out quite as Linda expected: 'Although I did slim down, mainly by cutting down on everything I enjoyed, I found it very hard indeed to keep the weight off. Then, twelve years after Vicky's birth, I found I was pregnant again with my third daughter Emma who's now eight. After she was born, I got fatter and fatter and I despaired of ever looking good again.'

Poor Linda hid her bulges under an all-concealing 'uniform' consisting of a size 18 black skirt, T-shirt and boots, and hated socialising.

'I joined the Fatfield group at the very beginning in January 1991,' she says. 'I went on the Steady Weight Loss Plan for six weeks, and lost over a stone. 'I felt confident enough to wear a swimsuit, and joined the Aquafit class at the Washington Leisure Centre near Fatfield.'

She has now maintained her weight of 9st 7lb for nearly two years, by following the Fatfield Maintenance Plan.

'I have loads more confidence these days, and have become a real exercise fan. When I finish work, I feel quite tired but I find that a stepping or Aquafit session gives me renewed energy.

'I now think very carefully about what I eat. As I work surrounded by food all day, I make sure that I am very selective about what I choose for myself and my family. I always stick within the Fatfield principles.'

On a typical day, Linda tucks into a cereal and fruit breakfast, a tuna salad and roll for lunch, then a large, cooked evening meal. She snacks on fruit, drinks plenty of water and allows herself an occasional glass of wine.

Emma now joins her mum for swimming and Aquafit, and Linda's two grandchildren Tony, three, and two-year-old Adele, are delighted with their energetic granny.

At the Fatfield Christmas Party last December, Linda presented me with her old black size 18 skirt which is now one of our favourite Fatfield 'museum pieces', along with her enormous size 18 Bermuda shorts (pictured on the back cover of the book)!

She weighs in every week at our Fatfield pub, the Biddick Inn, along with her friends and neighbours. 'Although I am a lot older than some of Emma's friends' mums, I do look about the same age. 'People who say you can't beat the age barrier should try the Fatfield Diet. It's a youth tonic!'

CHAPTER SEVEN

HOW TO STICK TO YOUR DIET

Is your willpower so wobbly that you fear that you will go *off* your diet within a few days of starting it? If so, you must realise that it is vital to prepare yourself mentally to lose weight. It is not an easy thing to do and I get very angry with those who throw scorn at overweight people, calling them 'greedy' or 'fat slobs'. Frankly, I have met very few greedy fat slobs in my time. Almost every overweight person we have counselled over the years has had a very good reason for putting on the pounds. Maybe they have had children in rapid succession, and found it difficult to shape up between pregnancies, or maybe they have had an illness which has made them unable to take exercise. Very often, there are emotional reasons why both men and women overeat. I cannot accept that emotional food cravings are a purely feminine problem. We have worked with many, many men who eat, and drink, too many of the wrong things because they are suffering from stress, depression, or sexual problems. Fat is a human issue, not just a feminist one.

If you are to win the battle of the bulge, you need four important things: the right diet plan, motivation, imagination, and lots of support. Well, you have definitely found the right diet plan, so now let's look at the other three factors:

MOTIVATION

Do have a long, hard think about the *reason* why you want to lose weight. At our first meeting with the Fatfield slimmers, three main reasons emerged. The first two were pretty general: everyone wanted to improve their health and appearance.

There were men like John Herkes who had already given up smoking, put on a bit of weight, and now wanted to be slim and trim as well as free of his nicotine addiction. Then, there was brave Erika Lowdon, who faced serious surgery and wanted to be in top form to help her recover swiftly. Lovely Rose Irwin (who lost 28lb altogether) vowed that she wanted to look good in hot pants and wear them to church to amaze the vicar!

But most of our slimmers had another, strong personal reason for wanting to lose weight too: such as pretty Yvette Bainbridge who wants to look slim on her wedding day later this year (she has already lost over 4 stone); or Dave Jameson, who had neglected his diet while unemployed and wanted to get back into shape; and his wife, Julie, who was plagued by health problems and realised that shedding weight would help her – both physically and psychologically. They all managed to achieve these aims by their own brilliant efforts.

Consider these ten good, medical reasons for losing those excess pounds:

1. *Lengthen your life*. It is sad but true that fat people die younger than slim people. According to data collected by the insurance companies, there is a direct connection between early mortality and excess weight. The odds are shortened if you are what is clinically termed 'obese' – that is around 20 per cent overweight.

2. *Beat heart disease*. The fatter you are, the greater the

risk of dying of a heart attack. Your heart has to work harder pumping blood around your body and the level of cholesterol in your arteries increases. So there is a far greater chance of arteries becoming blocked, and your poor old heart giving up the struggle!

3. *Lower your blood pressure.* High blood pressure increases your chances of having a heart attack or a stroke – both can be fatal. If you lose weight, you stand a very good chance of having normal blood pressure levels, which is more fun than taking tablets all your life and constantly living in fear of serious illness.

4. *Prevent aches and pains.* Joint problems such as arthritis and rheumatism are made much worse if you are overweight. The extra pressure makes your joints work harder and they are therefore more likely to wear out. Imagine carrying a couple of 10lb bags of potatoes everywhere – that is what your poor old hips, knee joints and feet have to put up with even if you are merely 1 stone 6lb overweight.

5. *Breathe more easily.* Do you wheeze, cough, and splutter as you struggle upstairs? Have you given up trying to climb up to the top deck of the bus? Do you catch all the colds going every winter? Maybe your lungs are fed up with trying to function properly surrounded by so much flab.

6. *Avoid diabetes.* One type of diabetes occurs in middle or old age, and is triggered by overweight. Controlling it requires patience, a special diet, tablets, or even regular insulin injections. It has been estimated that thousands of fat people are diabetics without realising it, feeling run down and ill all the time.

7. *Make surgery easier*. However fit you are, there are times when surgery can be necessary. If a surgeon has to cut through layers of fat to do a routine operation, then complications become far more likely. Post-operative care takes much longer and recovery is slowed down.

8. *Reduce the risk of infertility*. If you are fat, you reduce your chances of conceiving a baby easily. Fat people who attend infertility clinics are advised to slim down. In any case, it is always wise to get into good shape, and eat a healthy diet before conception, to ensure that your baby has a perfect start.

9. *Beat digestive complaints*. These can vary in seriousness from indigestion, gassiness and pain – all caused by overloading the stomach – to complaints such as gall bladder disease and gall stones which occur more frequently in overweight people.

10. *Enjoy an active sex life*. A loving sex life is good for your health. While there is no doubt that overweight people can have just as much fun in bed as slim people, it is a fact that you feel better about yourself when you are slim. That means you are less likely to be inhibited about sex and more likely to get your fair share and, even more important, to enjoy it!

Now check out these ten cost-cutting reasons for losing weight:

1. Large-size clothes cost more than normal, off-the-peg styles.

2. Cleaning bills mount up when you are fat because you perspire more, and need to change outfits more often.

3. Life insurance policies are expensive if you are huge and unhealthy.

4. Shoes wear out quickly when they are carrying 15 stone of flab around all day long.

5. Car seats and suspension take a bashing when they come into daily contact with a massive bum!

6. Food bills mount up if you are consuming high-calorie foods like cakes, puddings and sweets. The Fatfield Diet is designed to fit in with a family budget.

7. Household wear-and-tear is maximised when there is a large person in the house, flopping on the sitting-room sofa and bouncing on the bed.

8. It is unfair but true that 'fatties' are less likely to get promotion at work than slim people.

9. Holidays become expensive when you have to fork out extra cash for supersized swimsuits and beachwear.

10. You use a lot more of everyday items like washing powder, body lotion, deodorant and soap. Little things do add up!

Most important of all, think positive. Here are five very personal reasons for losing weight, contributed by the Fatfield slimmers. You probably have some of your own. Make a list for yourself.

1. 'I want to wear a red basque and a tight skirt to a party.' (*Linda Philpott*)

2. 'I want to feel fit enough to exercise, have a career *and* look after my family.' (*Vera Churnside*)

3. 'I want to look terrific when I launch my book about my son, Craig.' (*Marion Shergold*)

4. 'I'm going to look marvellous on my wedding day.' (*Yvette Bainbridge*)

5. 'I'm going to improve my running technique, and achieve some faster times.' (*Alison Wilkinson*)

IMAGINATION

It may be a long, long time since you were slim. So, it is hard to picture yourself looking any other shape than you are right now. But, one of the most helpful things you can do during your slim-in is to imagine yourself slim.

Psychologists have found that mental attitude can make or break your slimming campaign. By having your mind 'tuned in' to your new image, it will help your body to conform to *that* image. If this sounds far-fetched, let me tell you that most slimmers who succeed in losing large amounts of weight are those who have a very clear idea of how they might look and behave as slim people. Sometimes, this 'body-image awareness' does not register straight away, but an event, picture in a magazine, or chance remark from a friend triggers it off, so the slimmer has a sudden realisation of just what he or she might look like once the stones and pounds have dropped off. Once that picture is firmly lodged in the brain, bingo! – the diet starts to work.

A good example of this is one of our Fatfield brides, Julie Mulvaney. Julie, who is a play area assistant, would be the first to admit that she was struggling with her diet. She weighed in at $12^1/_2$ stone, and at the third weigh-in, she still weighed exactly the same. It was very puzzling indeed. She says, 'I could not see myself as a slim person. So, I cheated. My husband is a continental lorry driver and away for long periods, so I consoled myself by eating the wrong things. Then, I would miss out on meals – which goes right against the Fatfield Diet principles and is disastrous for someone like me who works, and eats, with children.' We organised a day in London for Julie, with a new hair-do and make-up. It gave her the chance to see a 'new' self.

Here are some 'mind over body' exercises *you* can do to help you tune in to the most powerful slimming aid of all, your brain:

1. Spend 10 minutes each day 'psyching' yourself slim. Lie down on a sofa or couch, close your eyes, and breathe regularly for a few moments. Let your mind wander, with different images flitting in and out of your brain. Now focus on an image of yourself, looking slim and fit, in a familiar situation – perhaps at a party, walking along a favourite beach, or entertaining friends at home. You are feeling good, the atmosphere is happy, people are laughing. Keep that image firmly in your mind for a few minutes. Then just relax and let your mind wander again. Every day 'tune in' to that person – he or she is *you*!

2. Let your imagination run riot when you read magazines and go to the cinema. Picture yourself in the glamorous clothes worn by the fashion models or the actors. Imagine yourself in exciting situations. Things only happen if you allow yourself to believe that it is a possibility that they might.

3. Take a fresh look at yourself. Julie had a 'make-over' – you can too. Have a new hair-cut, get some advice on make-up, ask your closest friends how they see you. If you are overweight, the chances are that you dress conservatively. It isn't necessary to do so. Don't wait until you are reed-slim, revamp your wardrobe now by buying one or two cheap bright items.

SUPPORT

The Fatfield slimmers were lucky because they had the support of friends, relatives, myself and my assistant, Toni, during their slimming and fitness campaign. The village, and surrounding area, is full of warm, charming people who love to get together. Families like John, Anne and Debbie Herkes encouraged each other to stay the course. Relatives like Julie Mulvaney and her sister-in-law Vera Churnside, provided mutual support. Whole groups of slimmers turned out to events like aquarobics sessions at the local pool and aerobics and weight-training classes.

At every weigh-in, there was a family party atmosphere. Slimmers were encouraged to bring friends and children along too. While advice was given privately if needed, slimmers could also involve their husbands and wives in the proceedings if they wished. There were strictly no penalties for not losing weight, just bags of encouragement all the way. One of the most important pieces of advice we gave our slimmers was to aim *low*: to think about the first half-stone, then the next . . . and so on.

Although it is obviously a tremendous advantage, and highly unusual, to get this degree of help while you slim, there are other ways to get support. Here are some ideas:

1. *Slim with your partner*. If you help your husband, wife or lover to lose a stone or two, and do the same yourself, it will strengthen your relationship. Be strong for them when their willpower wavers, praise their success, and take regular exercise together. Aim to be a glamorous, slim couple on that next holiday abroad, or for a special night out. It is important to be positive, so never nag!

2. *Slim with some friends*. Form a group – at work, with neighbours, or at the pub. Get together, follow the

Fatfield Diet, and raise some cash for a local good cause. It will be great fun and make the going easier. It is important to make sure that all group members check with their doctors before joining in.

3. *Be your own Slimming Counsellor*. If you prefer to go it alone, you can still get loads of encouragement – from yourself. Be your own best friend throughout your slim-in. Weigh yourself once a week, on the same scales, and keep a record of your progress. Keep that awful old photograph of yourself in an album, and get a friend to take regular Polaroid snaps of the new, emerging you. Gloat unashamedly at the improvement. Reward yourself with a new paperback, a trip to the cinema, or a couple of hours spent listening to music.

4. *Join our Fatfield Slim Pals*. While we were helping the Fatfield slimmers, we established a nationwide network of slimmers who keep in touch with each other by letter and telephone. We have matched up people with similar problems, so they can be mutually supportive. In some cases, our Slim Pals have met, exchanged views on slimming, and become firm friends. If you think you would benefit from chatting or writing to someone who is trying to lose weight, write to me at the address below, enclosing a stamped, addressed envelope and brief details about yourself, and your weight problems. We will send you full details about the Bazaar Slim Pals scheme.

Write to: Fatfield Slim Pals, c/o Sally Ann Voak, PO Box 618, Coulsdon, Surrey, CR5 1RU.

CHAPTER EIGHT

THE FATFIELD WORKOUT

We all know that exercise is good for us but most of us are too lazy to get out of our armchairs and go jogging, swimming or even for a brisk walk. Despite the boom in exercise tapes and videos, fitness classes, and sports clubs, the vast majority of people would still rather read about people exercising, or watch them doing it on television, than work out themselves. There are many overweight, unfit people who boast a whole shelf full of exercise videos, but have never tried to follow any of them.

Back in January 1991, when we started our fitness campaign, the residents of the little village of Fatfield were, like most of us, keen on thinking about exercise, but not so keen on doing any. But as the weight dropped off, they became much more fitness-conscious. Luckily for them, they had a highly qualified local fitness teacher, Susan Collins, to guide them. Susan runs classes in just about every form of exercise, from aquarobics to weight-training. Her base is the local community centre, and her classes are reasonably priced and always great fun.

The experience of Fatfield has proved to me that the best way to exercise is to start gently with swimming, walking and sitting-down routines, and work up to more vigorous sessions as you improve. Indeed, if you are a very overweight person, it is essential to take things very easily at first. Even if you are only a stone or so above your ideal weight, it is madness to leap into a vigorous aerobics class or go for 4-mile jogs every night if you are not used to it. You will end up with pulled muscles, possible back troubles, injuries to your joints or even a heart attack.

Our slimmers began with gentle aquarobics (exercises in water), swimming, simple stretching exercises, isometrics (exercises where the muscle is contracted through pushing, pulling, squeezing or pressing against an immovable object), and 'couch potato' exercises performed while watching television. Some found that they obtained a good level of fitness for their lifestyle with just one or two of the above. Some progressed to aerobics sessions, and even weight-training. I am proud to say that a few became so fit that they managed to survive a gruelling army assault course.

I have to admit that the Fatfield slimmers put me to shame. I gave up trying to fit exercise classes into my life some time ago, but I have always done isometric and 'couch potato' exercises while I work and watch television, and I try to break off work for a few stretching exercises a couple of times a day. I walk for miles at weekends, and occasionally treat myself to a course of toning table exercises, which are very effective indeed and involve the minimum of time and effort. In just one hour, you relax on six or eight different mechanical tables, which make your muscles work fairly hard while you simply breathe and move correctly. You feel refreshed afterwards but you do not look dishevelled and the inches do gradually come off, especially if you combine the course with one of the Fatfield diet plans.

The amount of fun obtained from exercise is of paramount importance. It is no earthly good doing any fitness routine unless you enjoy it. You may shape up your body but you are also likely to develop a harassed expression, frown lines, a droopy chest and a terrible passion for comfort foods.

Here are five great routines for lazy people like me and the Fatfield slimmers. They are all very easy, take up little time, and (most important) are safe for people on a slimming diet. At the end of the day, there really is no point in being super-fit unless you are an Olympic athlete. It is much better to achieve a level of fitness that helps you cope with the demands of your own lifestyle and guards against heart disease. That means you need a brisk workout three times a week which lasts 20 minutes, or longer, plus individual exercises to tone up the bits of you that wobble about.

AQUAROBICS AND BATH EXERCISES

Water is the ideal medium for exercise, especially if you are tense or tired, recovering from illness or injury, or are overweight.

It helps you exercise in two important ways: first, the pressure of water against your body (its resistance) helps you to build up strength gradually – you have to exert your muscles to get through the water. Second, its buoyancy supports the weight of your body, relieving the pressure of gravity on your spine and allowing the muscles of your legs and back (which usually have to work very hard to keep you standing up) to relax.

If you are a 'plumpie' who is shy about revealing your body in a swimsuit, you can either go to the pool in the early morning or throw caution to the wind and join a class.

Our intrepid Fatfield slimmers found that the hilarity of one of Susan's classes made them forget their wobbles and just have fun. If you can find a similar class in your area, do go along and join in – you could find that there are many people who are a lot fatter than you.

Try these in your local pool:

1. *Warm-up* Have a good splash about to get your circulation going. At waist-depth, jump repeatedly in all directions. Fling out your arms when you are at the top of the jump and keep your tummy muscles taught throughout.

2. *For spine, ankles, legs* With the water at waist level or deeper, face the side of the bath and hold it with both hands, about 3 feet (1 metre) apart. Now, let your legs float up behind you and kick without letting your feet break the surface of the water, keeping your knees straight, and taking very small 'steps'. Repeat 10 times, increasing to 25.

3. *For chest, back, shoulders, arms* Stand in shoulder-depth water and extend your arms together in front of you, then pull them back to the open-arm position. Try to get your shoulder blades to touch at the back and keep your fingers open for maximum 'drag'. Repeat 10 times, increasing to 25.

4. *For waist, side muscles, thighs, knees, arms* Stand with your feet wide apart in midriff-depth water. Now let your arms float on top of the water in front of you, and twist to the left and the right from your waist, using your arms as 'oars', and going as far as is comfortable with each swing. Repeat 10 times, increasing to 25.

5. *For bottom, hips and thighs* Stand waist-deep in the water, with legs comfortably apart, hands on your hips.

Jump to bring your feet together. Repeat 5 times, increasing to 20, when you get the hang of it.

6. *For legs, posture, balance* Still with water at waist-level, raise your hands straight out in front of you, palms down, and walk backwards through the water for a few steps. Walk forwards again. Repeat 5 times, trying to keep your balance and posture perfect.

Try these movements in the bath
You will get the same advantages as you do with aquarobics in the pool, with the added bonus of being able to do the exercises nude and in private. A bath pillow is essential, so you can relax while you work out.

1. *For tummy, thighs and lower back muscles* Lie back in the bath, arms by your sides, feet together, head resting comfortably on the bath pillow. Now, slowly raise your arms to the horizontal position, bending your knees and raising your feet off the bottom of the bath at the same time. Point your toes, hold the position for a count of 6, then lower feet and arms slowly. Repeat 5 times, increasing to 10.

2. *For tummy, legs, hips, shoulders, arms* Lie back in the bath, legs stretched out and toes wedged firmly under the taps, hands by your sides. Sit up slowly and stretch your arms to try and touch your toes, gently curl forward so your face comes down towards the water if you can. Hold for a count of 3, then relax back slowly. Repeat twice, increasing to 6 times.

3. *For tummy* Lie back again, feet resting on the bottom of the bath, knees bent, hands floating by your sides. Now pull in your tummy muscles, almost as though you were trying to touch your spine with your navel. Hold for a

113

count of 3 then relax. Repeat 5 times, resting between each exercise. Breathing is important here: breathe out deeply before you pull in your tummy muscles, breathe in again as you release them.

4. *For waist* Sit up in the bath, resting your feet on the bottom, legs slightly apart. Clasp your hands behind your head, making sure your back is straight, head held high. Twist your trunk slowly to the right, going as far as is comfortably possible. Hold for a count of 3, then return to starting position, and relax for a further count of 3. Repeat, twisting to the left this time. Repeat the whole movement 10 times.

WALKING

Walking just has to be the most underestimated form of exercise. It is free, easy, enjoyable and something we all do (although some of us try to avoid it as much as possible). Yet, it has never really caught on as a serious form of exercise.

Regular walking really can do a great deal to help you slim down and shape up your body. For a start, it uses up energy in a positive way. While you are walking, you are burning off calories at the rate of about six a minute. That might not sound much but it soon adds up. What's more, walking 'revs' up your metabolism and helps you burn off calories more quickly. This effect carries on, even when you stop walking. Contrary to what most people imagine, walking suppresses hunger pangs so, unless you plan your daily excursion to take in the local baker's, sweetshop, and fish and chip shop, you will be less likely to eat the wrong foods. It also gives you the mental relaxation you need to combat problems like stress and depression, which can also make you eat the wrong things.

Most important, walking makes you physically healthier and improves your looks by reducing fat and adding lean tissue at the same time. Some years ago, an interesting American study compared three groups of women. The first group cut back their daily food intake by 500 calories. The women in the second group ate the same amount as usual, but took enough exercise to burn off 500 calories daily. The third group did half and half, cutting back on 250 calories daily, and taking enough exercise to burn off another 250. The exercisers all worked out by walking on a treadmill. At the end of 16 weeks, the women had all lost roughly the same amount of weight, between $10^1/_2$ and $12^1/_2$lb each. But, the women who had taken exercise reshaped their bodies – losing more body fat (about $12^1/_2$lb) and gaining lean tissue. So, if you want your diet to work brilliantly and you also want to look firmer and leaner afterwards, follow the Fatfield Diet and *walk* your way to fitness. Here are six ways to do it:

1. *Leave the car at home*. You really do not need to drive to the corner shop, or to visit a friend a couple of streets away. It is a pleasure, more environmentally aware, and often quicker, to walk. Aim for a brisk, half-hour walk every single day.

2. *Choose an interesting spot*. Select a fascinating stretch of town, or a pretty walk in the country to be your very own walking route. Time yourself as you walk it, aiming to increase your pace from the normal human walking pace of between 3 and 4 miles an hour.

3. *Wear comfortable shoes*. You will never enjoy walking if your feet are killing you. Wear well-fitting sports shoes or trainers with good arch and ankle support, or low-heeled shoes or boots that do not rub or pinch.

4. *Walk with a friend*. It doesn't matter whether your chum is a lover, dog, or child, you will both get a big kick out of walking together, away from the pressures of your family, work or television set.

5. *Step out indoors*. Crazy though it sounds, you probably do most of your walking inside your own home. The trouble is that normally you do not walk briskly enough for it to do very much good. Try hotting up the action, by dashing up and down stairs, walking on the spot while you watch a lunchtime television show, or even using the bottom step of the stairs for some 'stepping'. This is the hot 'new' exercise rave in America, and simply consists of stepping up and down on a portable platform. Your own front doorstep is just as good.

6. *Be a happy hiker*. The cheapest way to have fun at weekends is to take a bus into the country, and go for a ramble. It may sound old-fashioned but it does wonderful things for your shape and for your bank balance. What's more, you see something of the countryside, instead of just whizzing through it in a car. All you need are stout shoes, a hooded waterproof jacket and some low-calorie sandwiches from your Fatfield Diet plan.

ISOMETRICS

If you want to work your muscles hard without any huffing and puffing, try these exercises. They are isometrics, and the muscle is contracted through pushing, pulling, squeezing or pressing against an immovable object. The force of resistance acts as pressure and the muscle is made to work very hard, promoting strength, tone and endurance.

The beauty of these exercises is that you can do them at home, at work, or even while travelling.

1. *For inside thigh muscles* Sit comfortably with your back straight and shoulders relaxed. Now place a suitably sturdy object such as a briefcase or metal wastepaper basket, between your feet. Squeeze your feet together as hard as possible for a count of 10, then relax. Repeat 10 times.

2. *For upper arms* Sit with your back straight, feet together, shoulders relaxed, and place the palms of your hands on a table or desk in front of you. Now press down as hard as you can, as if you were trying to force the table down. Hold the position for a count of 6. Relax. Now put your hands just under the table, palms up, elbows tucked in. Push up as hard as you can, hold for a count of 6, then relax. Repeat each movement 5 times.

3. *For upper back and tummy muscles* Sit with your back straight, feet slightly apart, palms of your hands flat on your thighs. Keeping your arms perfectly straight, take a breath, then exhale as you press down, pulling in your tummy muscles at the same time. Hold for a count of 6, then relax. Inhale and repeat 5 times.

4. *For chest muscles* Sitting in your car (while parked!) or at your desk, grip the steering wheel at the nine o'clock and three o'clock positions or place the palms of your hands against the sides of your computer terminal or typewriter. Now push hard with elbows tucked in (women should see their bosom 'jump' slightly), hold for a count of 6, then relax. Repeat 5 times.

COUCH POTATO EXERCISES

If you watch television for three or four hours every evening, it makes sense to combine your viewing with some easy exercises. Do them during the boring bits, or the commercials. It is a good idea to sit on a firm chair for one of the exercises, although you can do most of them sitting on the sofa.

1. *For shoulders* Sit with your back straight, feet slightly apart, hands clasped loosely behind you with elbows slightly bent. Now draw your shoulder blades together, and push your upper arms together, without trying to straighten your arms. Repeat 6 times.

2. *For bottom* Sit with your back straight, feet slightly apart and forward with knees slightly bent. Place the palms of your hands on your upper chest and relax your shoulders. Now contract your thigh muscles hard, and rotate them outwards. You should feel your buttock muscles contracting. Relax and repeat 6 times.

3. *For waistline* Sit with your back straight, the palms of your hands on your upper chest. Now lift your breastbone and rib-cage and twist your torso and head around to the left as far as you can with your pelvis still facing forwards. Now twist just a little more in short, sharp movements. Return to face the front and repeat to the right. Repeat 6 times each way.

4. *For tummy and pelvis* Sit near the front of a straight-backed chair for this one. Your feet should be flat on the floor, knees slightly apart, and you should grasp the seat of the chair near the back. Now, keeping your back straight, inhale, then exhale as you tilt your pelvis up so the pubic bone rises but your bottom stays put, in a rolling movement. The curve of your lower spine will straighten and your tummy will be pulled in. Relax and repeat 10 times.

5. *For bust* Sit with your knees slightly apart, shoulders relaxed, back straight. Now clench your fists and bring your arms upwards strongly, elbows bent, so they cross

over in front of you. Repeat this 'scissors' movement 20 times.

6. *For legs* Sorry, for this one you have got to get off the sofa and lie down on the carpet, but you can still carry on watching your favourite programme. Lie on your right side with your body and legs in a straight line. Prop your head on your right hand with your left hand on the floor in front of you for balance. With your foot flexed (the toe pointing forwards), raise your leg as high as you can comfortably do so. Pause briefly, then lower it to about 10 inches off the floor. Repeat 5 times, swap sides and repeat. (While you are facing away from the television set, get your family to fill you in on the action!)

STRETCHING EXERCISES

These are excellent exercises to do in the middle of the day, or when you get home from work. They help you unwind your body, particularly if it has been confined behind a bench, desk or driving wheel all day long. It is essential to do them in a warm room, wearing loose clothing, and to start off very gently. These six exercises are based on yoga *asanas* which are wonderful for helping to banish stress, improve concentration, and relieve depression and anxiety. I do recommend slimmers to try yoga, particularly those who eat the wrong things when they are under pressure.

1. *Relaxation* Lie on your back on the floor with your legs slightly apart, hands a little way from your body, palms uppermost. Now, let your feet flop open and close your eyes, breathing quietly and evenly. Allow yourself two or three minutes of complete relaxation, then open your eyes, and get up slowly.

2. *For tummy and thighs* Kneel with your back straight, head erect and arms relaxed beside you. Take a deep breath, and hold it as you lean back, making sure your body and thighs stay in a straight line. Go just a little way at first. Hold for a count of 2 then straighten up smoothly, breathing in as you do so. Repeat 4 times, then relax, sitting back on your heels.

3. *For spine, shoulder and neck muscles* Kneel on the floor and place your hands on the floor in front of you with hands shoulders' width apart. Breathing slowly and normally throughout the movement, hollow your back and look up at the ceiling. Count to 5, then reverse the position by arching your back and gently pushing your pelvis forward. Try to make your chin touch your chest. Count to 5 and repeat the entire movement twice. Rest, sitting back on your heels for a few moments, then repeat twice more.

4. *For spine, tummy and chest* Lie on your tummy on the floor. Bend your elbows and place the palms of your hands in front of you, fingertips touching, so you can rest your left cheek on the backs of your hands. Now take a breath and exhale as you press your hands down, straighten your arms and raising your upper body off the ground. Look up at the ceiling, count to 5, and relax down to the first position, breathing in as you do so. Repeat 3 times.

5. *For legs and ankles* Stand straight, head erect, legs and feet together. Now raise your arms in front of you to shoulder level, palms of your hands facing the floor. Keeping your back perfectly straight, take a breath, then exhale as you bend your knees and come up onto the balls of your feet. Go down as far as possible without wobbling. Now breathe in as you straighten up. Repeat 4 times.

6. *For back, legs, arms, tummy muscles* Stand, feet together, arms above your head, fingers clasped loosely.

Look up at your hands. Bend your knees and bring your hands down slowly to the horizontal position, with your knees bent. Let your hands fall sideways and down, and relax your head forward, bending your knees still further. Pause, then reverse the movement. Repeat 5 times. Breathe in as you raise your body, out as you lower it.

CHAPTER NINE

HOW TO KEEP WEIGHT OFF – THE FATFIELD WAY

One very important effect of the Fatfield Diet is that, once you stop slimming, weight does *not* creep back on easily. You really have to work at it!

Joking aside, it is quite difficult to eat much more than you are already eating on the diet. After you have tasted so much good, healthy, enjoyable food, it takes time to slip back into old habits. Fatty foods seem greasy and disgusting, over-cooked vegetables look unappetising, sugar in your tea tastes just awful. The diet re-trains your eating habits so well that you do not want to rush for a cream bun 'fix' as soon as you reach your goal weight.

It is well known that many slimming plans encourage you to put weight back on when you stop dieting. After weeks, or months of deprivation, your body is delighted when extra food arrives on the scene and promptly stores it – as fat. On the Fatfield Diet, calories are never cut down too much, and bulk is maintained all the way through. The result? Satisfaction not deprivation.

It is still too early to say whether all our Fatfield slimming guinea-pigs will keep off the weight they have lost on the diet. Several did reach their 'goal' during the slim-in and have kept off the weight very successfully indeed since then. One reason for this is that they all learned to enjoy exercising while they dieted and have kept up regular work-outs ever since. This helps keep their metabolism in 'top gear', so the fuel-burning processes have not become sluggish.

They also enjoyed the feeling of well-being produced by eating healthy foods instead of fat or sugar-loaded 'junk' food.

'I never imagined that I would enjoy exercise so much,' says Linda Philpott, 'or that I would be able to fit it into my life.' Linda works in a busy supermarket and has a young daughter to look after. Yet somehow she manages to go swimming and weight-training, and lead a hectic social life. 'Before I lost weight, I'd wake up tired and be too tired at the end of the day to do a thing except watch television. Now, I have so much energy.'

Lynn Ayre, who was the first slimmer to shed 2 stone, and now weighs 11 stone 10lb, says, 'The big moment for me came when I bought a clingy, black Lycra dress in a size 14. It was the first time I had worn size 14 since my wedding day ten years ago. As soon as I put it on, and looked in the mirror, I vowed that I would *never* get fat again – and I won't!'

When you feel as good as that about yourself, it is crazy to go off the straight and narrow. But, guess what, I am now going to give you permission to do just that. Eating the wrong things, occasionally, is not a sin. What is important is how you deal with it. It is also important to find out just how many calories you can consume without putting on weight. The Fatfield Maintenance Plan on page 127 has been specially devised to help you work out your own best calorie intake level.

It gives a good basic diet, allowing about 1500 calories for women, 1800 for men. Follow it for two weeks after you finish your Fatfield Slimming Diet plan, and weigh in at the end of the two weeks. If you are still losing, add one of the 100 calorie Extras (which include sweet treats, more bread, and even a little more alcohol) to the plan and follow it for one more week.

If the pounds are still dropping off, add another 100 calorie Extra, follow the diet for a further week – and so on.

When you have established the perfect calorie level to maintain your weight, try to stick within that range. If you consume more calories one day, try to make up for it the next day by eating simple, healthy meals from our recipe section or the Basic Fatfield Plan with lots of green vegetables.

Here are your *Top Ten Rules* for staying in shape:

1. *Don't* panic if the scales show you have put on a few pounds. This could be caused by fluid retention, or a little over-indulgence. Calmly, go back on the basic Maintenance Diet, until the extra weight drops off again. At the same time, increase the amount of exercise you take. Just walking for an extra half-hour a day should do the trick.

2. *Don't* feel guilty if you eat chocolate, sweets or cakes. If you buy them furtively and wolf them down in secret, you will get a severe attack of guilt, which will make you crave *more* and could even lead to bingeing. Instead, enjoy your treat, eating it slowly and savouring every single mouthful. Make a mental note of the calories the treat contains and make sure you trim off the same amount from your next day's calorie total.

3. *Do* throw out your old clothes or alter them to fit your new shape. If you keep a wardrobe which consists of 'fat' and 'thin' outfits, you are programming yourself, mentally,

to pile on pounds again. Remember, you are a slim person now, so you do not need large-size clothes any more.

4. *Don't* eat too little. You might be tempted to slip back into bad old habits like eating very little during the first half of the day, then snacking all evening. It is very dangerous indeed to do this. Concentrate on maintaining a healthy food intake at all times.

5. *Do* show off your new body. It is very hard to become adjusted to a new, slim shape. Increase your self-confidence by going out and about much more than you did when you were fatter. Go for those goals we talked about on page 101. Wear shorts, join a hang-gliding club, sunbathe in a tiny swimsuit. Get your partner or a friend to take some good photographs of you, so you can keep your own *Before and After* record of your slimming achievement. Vanity is healthy, so keep right on admiring yourself and even buy a few new mirrors so you can really enjoy the view.

6. *Do* keep busy. One of the best bits of advice for anyone who wants to stay slim is to be too busy – with work, hobbies, and projects – to crave high-fat and high-carbohydrate snacks. If you are working full-time, cram some fitness or vocational evening classes into the day. If you are working part-time or not at all, join a club, help with your favourite charity, or plunge yourself into a task like redecorating the house or landscaping the garden.

7. *Do* be extra loving to your partner. Some slimmers find that their 'other half', intentionally or unintentionally, tries to sabotage all their efforts to stay slim by encouraging them to eat and drink the wrong things. Don't forget that it can be very upsetting to watch a familiar, well-rounded loved one change into a slim, dynamic person.

Naturally, your partner is bound to feel threatened by the new you. Be strong; show lots of love and concern, but refuse to allow the saboteur to pile up cheesecake on your plate, or pour you another large Scotch. Don't forget, *you* (and *only* you) are in charge of your own body!

8. *Do* become a Fatfield Supercook. Collect recipes and meal ideas which will enlarge your repertoire of huge, satisfying, low-fat high-fibre meals. Even better, invest in a copy of *The Fatfield Recipe Book* (£3.99, also published by Michael O'Mara Books Limited), which contains over 100 delicious calorie-counted recipes for hungry slimmers. It's on sale at W.H. Smith and most good bookshops.

9. *Do* write and tell me how you are getting on. We want as much information as possible about the long-term success of the Fatfield Diet. So do drop me a line – with photographs if possible – to the address on page 108. Do enclose a stamped, addressed envelope.

10. *Do* tell your friends how you lost weight. The more you can spread the word about the Fatfield Diet, the better. Once you have built up a reputation as a successful slimmer, you will have all the more reason for staying slim. Encourage others to change their lives the Fatfield way; they'll thank you for it when they see the pounds dropping off and start to feel wonderful!

HEALTHY EATING IS A WAY OF LIFE

If you follow the Maintenance Plan on the next page, you'll have a blueprint for healthy eating – and for life. It contains all the goodies you need to help you stay slim, trim, and full of vitality.

You can adapt the plan to fit in with your life style so long as you shop and cook wisely following the advice in this book. You'll reap the rewards of good nutrition with extra energy, fewer health problems, and lots more fun!

THE FATFIELD MAINTENANCE PLAN

EVERY DAY $^3/_4$ pint (425ml) skimmed milk for your tea and coffee, unlimited water, mineral water and diet soft drinks. Use an artificial sweetener such as Hermestas instead of sugar.

MEN   Add 2 slices wholemeal bread or a medium wholemeal roll with a little low-fat spread, plus 1 glass dry wine or $^1/_2$ pint beer or lager.

FREE VEGETABLES   Choose them from the list on page 37.

CALORIES   About 1500 calories for women, 1800 for men. You may add calories (as explained above) by choosing items from the 100 calorie Extras list below.

BREAKFAST (choose *one*, packed if necessary)

- $^1/_2$ grapefruit, with sweetener, 1oz (25g) any unsweetened cereal with milk from allowance, 1 slice wholemeal toast topped with 2 tsp honey or marmalade
- 1 slice wholemeal toast with 1 size 3 poached egg, half 5oz (125g) can baked beans, 1 large banana
- 1 Shredded Wheat biscuit, milk from allowance, 1 carton Diet Ski yogurt, 1 slice wholemeal toast with a little low-fat spread, 1 apple or pear
- Sandwich of 2 slices wholemeal bread with filling of 1 cooked low-fat sausage, mustard or 1 tsp tomato ketchup, 1 apple or orange

- 1 medium wholemeal roll with filling of 1 rasher well-grilled back bacon, grilled tomatoes, 5 fl oz (125ml) unsweetened fruit juice, 1 satsuma
- 2oz (50g) unsweetened muesli, milk from allowance, 1 chopped apple, 1 small carton natural yogurt
- 1 pot Golden Wonder Pot Noodles, any flavour, a few grapes
- 1 slice wholemeal toast topped with small (7.6oz/215g) can Heinz Spaghetti in Tomato Sauce, grilled tomatoes, 1 small banana

LUNCHES (choose *one*)

Sandwich made with 2 slices wholemeal bread or a medium sized wholemeal or granary roll with one of the following fillings and accompaniments:

- 1oz (25g) any hard cheese, 1 Diet Ski yogurt, 1 banana
- 2oz (50g) lean ham or chicken (no skin), 1 mug Batchelors Slim a Soup, 1 apple, orange or pear
- 1 well-grilled low-fat sausage, 1 tsp sweet pickle, 1 carton Shape Fromage Frais
- 1 pot Shippam's Paste, any flavour, 1 small carton cottage cheese with pineapple
- 1 pot Shape Low-Fat Soft Cheese, any flavour, 1 Harvest Crunch Bar

Do not forget to pile on the 'free' salad and vegetables, either in your sandwich or roll, or as a separate dish, packed in a sealed container to keep it crisp.

OR

One meal chosen from this list:

- 1 slice of melon, 6oz (150g) any grilled or steamed white fish, 5oz (125g) jacket potato, 1 apple or pear

- 1 well-grilled beefburger, 3oz (75g) oven chips, 1 orange
- 2 slices wholemeal toast topped with one of the following: 1 small can (5oz/125g) baked beans, 1 small can Heinz Wholewheat Spaghetti in Tomato Sauce, 1 poached egg. Followed by 1 apple or orange, and 1 digestive biscuit
- 6oz (150g) jacket potato, topped with 4oz (100g) chopped cooked chicken with 1 tbsp low-calorie salad cream, 1 apple
- 1 large slice of melon, 10oz (250g) chicken leg (no skin) grilled or roast, 1 small wholemeal roll with a little low-fat spread

Please do not forget your 'free' vegetables and salad.

SUPPERS (choose *one*)

Any of the suppers in the Basic Plan on page 48, plus 1 apple, orange or small banana.

OR
One of these:

- Any Findus Lean Cuisine ready meal with 5oz (125g) jacket potato
- 1 can (6oz/150g) John West Pilchards in Tomato Sauce with 3oz (75g) mashed potato, made up with milk from allowance, 2 crispbreads with a little low-fat spread
- 1 portion Kentucky Fried Chicken, 1 portion coleslaw, 1 apple or orange
- 1 McDonald's Cheeseburger, or 6 Chicken McNuggets, regular orange juice
- $^1/_2$ thin crust medium pizza from a pizza restaurant or takeaway, 1 apple or orange to follow

- Restaurant meal of melon or clear soup, simply-cooked fish or lean meat (no sauces), medium jacket potato

TREATS (choose *one* each day)

- 1 extra apple or orange
- 1 Jaffa Cake
- 1 After Eight Mint
- 1 small wholemeal roll with salad filling
- 1 mug Batchelors Slim a Soup with 1 crispbread
- 1 Ferrero Rocher chocolate
- 1 Rowntree Rolo
- 1 Diet Ski yogurt, any flavour

ALCOHOL
You may have ¹/₂ pint beer, lager or stout, or 1 glass dry wine or sherry, or 2 pub-measure 'short' drinks with low-calorie mixers.

100 CALORIE EXTRAS

- 1 slice wholemeal bread with a little low-fat spread
- 2oz (50g) (no skin) chicken, or ham (lean only), or lean beef, lamb or pork. In practice, that is an extra *thin* slice at dinner or suppertime.
- 4oz (100g) poached or grilled white fish with no fat added, or 3oz (75g) shellfish, again cooked without fat or sauces
- 2oz (50g) chunk roast potato, or 3oz (75g) potato, mashed with milk from your allowance
- 4oz (100g) peas, beans or sweetcorn
- ¹/₂ pint beer, lager or stout, or 1 glass dry wine, or 2 pub-measure 'short' drinks with low-calorie mixers.

CHAPTER TEN

RECIPES

All the recipes used in the Fatfield Diet have been calorie-counted. Measurements are given in metric as well as imperial weights – work in either, but *not* both.

I think you will find that the dishes are tasty and filling in true Fatfield fashion. Please serve up main courses with plenty of 'free' vegetables. Bon Appetit!

NB Ingredients in these recipes are given in ounces and the nearest equivalent in grams. The exact metric conversion does not give easy working quantities so I have rounded these off to the nearest 25 grams (or millilitres). As I said earlier, a set of kitchen scales makes measuring more accurate, together with a graduated measuring jug (1 pint/575 ml) for liquids. All spoon measurements given are level.

STARTERS

CITRUS SALAD IN YOGURT DRESSING

This is light and delicious. A perfect summer starter, and a scrumptious breakfast too.

2 medium oranges
2 medium grapefruit
20 green grapes
2 tbsp finely chopped fresh mint leaves
1 carton Shape Natural Yogurt
mint sprigs and 1 kiwi fruit to garnish

1. Grate the zest from 1 orange. Place in a bowl.
2. Remove all peel and pith from the oranges and grapefruit and discard. Halve grapes and remove pips. Then, over the bowl, carefully cut between membranes to remove citrus fruit segments.
3. Add chopped mint and yogurt to the grated zest, oranges, grapefruit and grapes in the bowl. Leave in the refrigerator to marinate. Serve garnished with mint leaves and sliced kiwi fruit.

Serves 4. Calories per portion: 107

GREEK VEGETABLE SOUP

Tasty and filling, this makes a good starter for a dinner party and is excellent for a family supper too. The tangy taste makes you think of balmy Mediterranean nights eating out under the stars.

15fl oz (425ml) canned consommé
4oz (100g) frozen mixed vegetables
10fl oz (275ml) natural unsweetened yogurt
1 egg yolk
1 tbsp chopped fresh mint
grated zest of $1/2$ lemon

1. Heat the soup with the vegetables, cover and simmer for 10 minutes.
2. Beat the yogurt with the egg yolk and gradually stir in some of the hot soup. Return to the pan and mix well until hot, but not boiling.
3. Serve sprinkled with herbs and lemon zest.

Serves 4. Calories per portion: 76

TONI'S MACKEREL AND LEMON PATÉ

This tasty and normally high-calorie paté is delicious with crisp-breads or Nimble toast. Serve for breakfast, lunch or as a starter.

6oz (175g) fillet smoked mackerel
5.3oz (150g) carton Shape low-fat soft cream cheese
1 tbsp lemon juice

1 tsp creamed horseradish sauce
freshly ground black pepper

1.   Remove the skin and any bones from the mackerel. Mash all
the ingredients together with a fork for a rough paté, or mix
together with an electric mixer for a smooth paté.
2.   Divide into 4 individual bowls or ramekin dishes.

Serves 4. Calories per portion: 155

FRENCH ONION SOUP

*This very low-calorie soup is ideal to use as a 'filler'. Make up a
batch and have some before your supper or before you go out for the
evening—it helps to curb your appetite. Don't be put off by the bread
and cheese—it is low in calories. Really!*

1lb (450g) large onions, finely chopped
1 beef stock cube
1 pint (575ml) water
1 tbsp brandy (for special occasions)
4oz (100g) piece of French bread
1oz (25g) Edam cheese, grated

1.   Add the finely chopped onions to the water and stock cube,
bring to the boil, and cook until soft. Simmer for 20 minutes.
2.   Remove some of the onions and put the soup and the rest of
the onions through a blender. Return to the saucepan and heat
through with the brandy if using it.
3.   Divide into 4 bowls. Add the reserved onions to the soup.
4.   In each bowl, add a 1oz piece (25g) of French bread and
sprinkle with a quarter of the cheese. Place under the grill until
the cheese has melted and the bread is soaked with soup.

Serves 4. Calories per portion: 150

LUNCHTIME SPECIALS

STUFFED TOMATOES

*The large 'beef' tomatoes are ideal for this delicious lunch dish. It is
less fiddly to make than it sounds and very filling indeed. It's also a*

great starter for a dinner party: simply serve one tomato for each person on a bed of lettuce with a wedge of lemon.

6 large tomatoes
2oz (50g) brown rice, boiled and drained
4oz (100g) smoked mackerel fillet, skinned and flaked
1oz (25g) flaked almonds
1 tsp chopped parsley
salt and black pepper
pinch of tarragon

1. Slice the top off each tomato. Scoop the flesh into a bowl. Turn the shells upside down to drain.
2. Chop the flesh. Add the remaining ingredients and mix well.
3. Spoon into tomato 'shells' and replace the tops.
4. Serve on a bed of salad from 'free' list.

Serves 3. Calories per portion: 320

WHOLEMEAL ROLLS WITH TASTY FILLINGS
Here's a selection of filling ideas for lunchtime rolls. They all serve one, and the calorie count includes a 2oz (50g) roll.

SPICY BANANA
1 small ripe banana, peeled and mashed
1 tbsp natural low-fat yogurt
1 level tsp low-calorie apricot or strawberry jam
pinch of ground ginger

Combine all ingredients in a small bowl and spread on split roll.

Calories per portion: 225

SARDINE AND CELERY
2oz (50g) sardines in tomato sauce
1oz (25g) celery, finely chopped
3 drops Worcestershire sauce

Mash sardines in a bowl, and blend with the chopped celery and Worcestershire sauce. Spread on split roll.

Calories per portion: 235

PRAWN COCKTAIL

1oz (25g) peeled prawns
1 dsp low-fat natural yogurt
1 tsp low-calorie mayonnaise
¼ tsp tomato ketchup
1 drop tabasco sauce

Combine all ingredients in a small bowl and spread on cut roll.

Calories per portion: 195

FRENCH BREAD PIZZA

This is lovely if you have some friends coming for lunch.

1 French stick, split and cut into six pieces
1 tbsp tomato purée
2 tsp olive oil
1 onion, peeled and sliced
1 green pepper, de-seeded and chopped
1 x 7oz (200g) can tuna in brine, drained
3 tomatoes, sliced
3oz (75g) Edam cheese, grated

1. Spread the French bread pieces with tomato purée.
2. Cook onion and pepper gently in low-fat spread until soft.
3. Add tuna, broken into chunks. Stir and continue cooking until tuna is heated through.
4. Divide tuna mixture between bread pieces. Cover with tomato slices and sprinkle over the cheese.
5. Place under a hot grill until the cheese is melted and bubbly. Serve at once.

Serves: 6. Calories per portion: 310

SUPPERS
SPAGHETTI CARBONARA

This traditional Italian favourite has had its calories trimmed so that it is suitable for slimmers with a taste for something sumptuous.

10oz (275g) (dry weight) spaghetti
6 rashers streaky bacon
2oz (50g) Shape Mature type cheddar
2 size 3 eggs
$^1/_4$ pint (150ml) Shape Single

1. Cook the spaghetti in boiling salted water.
2. Thoroughly grill the bacon and chop roughly.
3. Grate the cheese and beat the eggs.
4. Drain the spaghetti and return to the pan away from the heat. Add the bacon, Shape Single, egg and most of the cheese. Stir well to coat the spaghetti—the heat of the spaghetti will cook the eggs. Place in a hot serving dish and sprinkle with the remaining cheese.

Serves 4. Calories per portion: 450

STEAK AND KIDNEY CASSEROLE

A hearty family supper dish, or a Sunday 'special', this has the traditional taste without the fatty bits!

12oz (350g) stewing steak
6oz (175g) kidney
$^1/_2$oz (15g) low-fat spread
1 large onion
8oz (225g) mushrooms
1 pint (575ml) beef stock
1 tsp tomato purée
dash Worcestershire sauce
salt and pepper
2oz (50g) (dry weight) rice per person

1. Discard all visible fat from the cubed steak and kidney and place in a casserole dish. Add the finely chopped onion and the mushrooms, beef stock, tomato purée, a dash of Worcestershire sauce and salt and pepper.
2. Cook in the oven at 170°C, 325°F or gas mark 3 until the beef is tender (about 2 hours).

3.   Cook the rice and serve with the casserole.

Serves 4.   Calories per portion: 375 (includes rice)

PORK PAPRIKA

The paprika, onion and yogurt add an exotic touch to these deli-cious pork chops. This is a good dinner party choice as it is very easy to prepare, yet looks spectacular.

4 lean boneless pork chops (about 6oz/175g each)
salt and pepper
1 onion, chopped
$^1/_2$ tbsp oil
1 tbsp paprika (or to taste)
$2^1/_2$oz (65g) canned tomato purée
5 fl oz (125ml) stock made from chicken stock cube
6oz (175g) small button mushrooms
10oz (275g) natural yogurt

1.   Heat oven to 180°C, 350°F, gas mark 4.
2.   Season pork chops and put under grill to seal on both sides. Remove from heat, cut off fat. Keep to one side.
3.   In a flameproof casserole, gently cook onion in oil until soft. Blend in paprika and cook for a further minute. Add tomato purée. Remove from heat and blend in stock.
4.   Return to heat and bring to the boil, stirring well. Taste and adjust seasoning. Add the pork chops. Cover and cook for 30 minutes or until meat is tender.
5.   Five minutes before end of cooking time, add the mush-rooms. Just before serving, spoon over the natural yogurt.

Serves 4. Calories per portion: 260

FISH CASSEROLE

Coley is reasonably priced, so this casserole is not too expensive— despite the shrimps! A favourite for parties, served with rice, salad and crusty bread.

$1^1/_2$lb (675g) cod or coley fillet

1 clove garlic, chopped
1 large onion, finely sliced
1 tbsp olive oil
$^1/_2$oz (15g) low-fat spread
4 courgettes, washed and sliced
4oz (100g) mushrooms, peeled and sliced
4 tomatoes, skinned and chopped
2 tbsp tomato purée
7fl oz (200ml) water
dried basil
2oz (50g) black olives
4oz (100g) prawns or shrimps, peeled
salt and freshly ground black pepper
1 tbsp chopped parsley and 4–8 slices lemon for garnish

1.   Gently fry garlic and onion in olive oil and low-fat spread until translucent.
2.   Add courgettes, mushrooms, tomatoes, tomato purée, water, and basil. Season to taste. Cover and simmer for about 15 minutes.
3.   Add olives and prawns.
4.   Place fish in a heavy saucepan or casserole and pour sauce over it. Cover and simmer for 15–20 minutes until the fish is cooked.
5.   Garnish with freshly chopped parsley and slices of lemon and serve with 3oz (75g) peas and 4oz (100g) mashed potato.

Serves 4. Calories per portion: 240

FATFIELD BUBBLE AND SQUEAK

This is one of the Fatfield village favourites and a good, low-calorie way of using up leftover vegetables. Great as a Monday night supper dish, served with a huge mixed salad.

8oz (225g) cooked greens
2lb (900g) cooked mashed potato
2 carrots, peeled and grated
1 large onion

pinch nutmeg
1 tsp sunflower oil
2 tbsp grated wholemeal breadcrumbs
1oz (25g) grated strong Cheddar cheese

1. Chop the cooked greens and mix with the cooked mashed potato.
2. Place the grated carrots, sliced onion, pinch of nutmeg, and a splash of water into a saucepan. Cover and cook over gentle heat for 4 minutes.
3. Stir into the mashed potato mixture, and season.
4. Heat 1 tsp sunflower oil in a non-stick frying pan over a medium heat, add the vegetable mixture and level the top. Cook over a medium heat until the underside is crisp and golden. When cooked place under a hot grill until the top is brown.
5. Sprinkle the wholemeal breadcrumbs, and the grated cheese over the top and grill again until it is golden brown.

Serves 4. Calories per portion: 300

FATFIELD SHEPHERD'S PIE

This pie is highly recommended by Rose Irwin, one of our successful Fatfield slimmers, who dishes this up for her family and herself. No-one ever complains about eating Mum's diet food!

8oz (225g) lean minced beef
2 large onions
$^1/_2$oz (15g) low-fat spread
2 tsps oil
1 large can (15oz/425g) baked beans
$^1/_4$ pint (150ml) beef stock
1lb (450g) potato, cooked and mashed

1. Brown the minced beef in its own fat and drain on kitchen paper. Transfer to a pie plate
2. Fry the chopped onions in the low-fat spread and oil. Transfer to the mince and mix in the can of baked beans, adding enough stock to make a moist consistency.

3.   Spread the mashed potato over the top, fluff up with a fork, bake in the oven for 40 minutes until golden. Serve with 'free' vegetables.

Serves 4. Calories per portion: 300

LIVER AND ONION GRAVY

Liver is never dry and boring served with this delicious onion sauce. If you like the liver pink inside, cut down the cooking time by a minute or so.

1 small onion, finely chopped
$^1/_4$ pint (150ml) beef stock
4oz (100g) lamb's liver
1 heaped tbsp skimmed milk powder
1 tsp cornflour

1.   In a large frying pan, fry the finely chopped onion until translucent. Add 2tbsp water and the beef stock cube and cook for 4 minutes.
2.   Cut the lamb's liver into $^1/_4$-inch slices. Place on top of onions. Cover and cook for 10 minutes or until liver is tender. Remove meat from pan and keep warm.
3.   Add the skimmed milk powder to the cornflour and mix with 5 tbsp water. Stir into onion mixture and bring to the boil. Pour onion sauce over the liver. Serve with plenty of 'free' vegetables.

Serves 1. Calories per portion: 300

PIQUANT MINCE WITH DISHY DUMPLINGS

Whoever heard of eating dumplings on a slimming diet? Well, this is no ordinary diet and these are no ordinary dumplings. They are boiling over with taste-appeal!

12oz (350g) lean mince
1 small onion, chopped
1 stick celery, thinly sliced
1 small carrot, diced

1 beef stock cube
2 tbsp tomato purée
dash Worcestershire sauce
1 bay leaf
Dumplings
3oz (75g) self-raising flour
pinch salt
1$\frac{1}{2}$oz (40g) vegetable suet

1.   Brown the mince in a non-stick pan and then drain off the fat. Place meat in a casserole dish.
2.   Add the thinly sliced celery, chopped onion and diced carrot to the casserole dish and mix with the minced beef.
3.   Dissolve the stock cube and tomato purée in 7fl oz (200ml) boiling water, and add to the casserole. Add the Worcestershire sauce and bay leaf. Cover and cook at 190°C, 375°F, gas mark 5 for 45 minutes.
4.   Sieve the self-raising flour with the salt and add the vegetable suet. Mix with enough water to make a firm dough. Shape into 4 dumplings and place on top of the meat. Cook for 25 minutes. Serve with 'free' vegetables.

Serves 4. Calories per portion: 320

BEEF WITH BEAN CASSEROLE

Kidney beans help 'bulk out' this casserole, so it is less expensive than it looks. You can prepare this in advance and it freezes well, too.

12oz (350g) lean, cubed braising or stewing steak
1 tbsp sunflower oil
1 onion, sliced
1 green pepper, de-seeded and sliced
$\frac{1}{2}$oz (15g) wholemeal flour
1 pint (575ml) beef stock
pinch dried herbs
1 large can (15oz/425g) red kidney beans

1. Fry the beef in the cooking oil. Add the sliced onion and green pepper and fry until golden brown.
2. Add the flour, stirring all the time. Gradually pour on the stock and herbs. Cover and simmer, stirring occasionally, for 2 hours.
3. Add the beans 15 minutes before the end of the cooking time. Serve with 'free' vegetables.

Serves 4. Calories per portion: 250

AUBERGINE CASSEROLE

It's important to measure out the oil carefully in this recipe, as the aubergine slices soak it up like a sponge! However, it is still reasonably low in calories.

2 medium aubergines
1½ tsp salt
2 tbsp corn or olive oil
4 small courgettes, washed, trimmed and cut into ¼-inch thick slices
2 medium onions, sliced
2 garlic cloves, crushed
8oz (225g) can chopped tomatoes
½ tsp cayenne pepper
1 tsp ground cumin
1 large can (15oz/425g) chick peas, drained

1. Peel aubergines and dice flesh, place pieces in a colander and sprinkle with 1 tsp salt, leave for 30 minutes. Drain on kitchen paper.
2. Heat half the oil in a non-stick pan and add chopped aubergine. Cook for 10 minutes until pieces are evenly browned on all sides. Drain well on kitchen paper and transfer with any cooking liquid to a large mixing bowl.
3. Heat remaining oil, and add onions and garlic to the pan and cook for 5–7 minutes until onions are soft but not brown.

4.   Add tomatoes, courgettes, rest of salt, cayenne pepper and cumin and stir well to mix. Cook for 3 minutes then add to the aubergine mixture.

5.   Stir in the chick peas. Transfer mixture to an ovenproof casserole and bake in a moderate oven until all vegetables are tender.

Serves 4. Calories per portion: 230

CURRY CREOLE

Why go out for a curry, when you can cook up this delicious low-calorie recipe at home? It is a vegetarian dish that meat-eaters will love too.

2 tbsp oil
2 medium onions, thinly sliced
1 garlic clove, crushed
1 green chilli, de-seeded and sliced
4 small courgettes, trimmed and cut into $^1/_4$-in slices
1 large red pepper, de-seeded and sliced
3 tomatoes, blanched, peeled and chopped
2oz (50g) canned pineapple chunks, drained
1 tsp ground coriander
$^1/_2$ tsp each ground cardamon, fenugreek and tumeric
$^1/_4$ tsp hot chilli powder
3 tbsp water
$^1/_2$ pint (275ml) vegetable stock
2 medium bananas, sliced
1-inch slice of creamed coconut

1.   Heat the oil in a large saucepan over moderate heat, then add onions, garlic, chilli, courgettes and red pepper. Cook, stirring occasionally for 10 minutes.

2.   Add tomatoes and pineapple and cook, stirring frequently, for 3 minutes.

3.   Combine spices with water in a small bowl to make a smooth paste. Stir into the fruit and vegetable mixture, then pour in the vegetable stock. Increase heat to high and bring stock to the boil.

Reduce heat to low, cover and simmer for 15 minutes or until vegetables are cooked. Add bananas.

4.   Stir in creamed coconut, mixing until it dissolves and the liquid thickens. Simmer for further 2 minutes, then transfer to a warmed dish and serve immediately.

Serves 4. Calories per portion: 270

CRUNCHY WHOLEWHEAT LASAGNE

Delicious and filling, this is a great choice for a Saturday family lunch, with dry white wine, crusty bread and plenty of green salad.

8oz (225g) lean minced meat
10oz (283g) can/jar Italian tomato sauce
$^1/_4$ pint (150ml) beef stock
3oz (75g) Gold low-fat spread
2oz (50g) flour
1 pint (575ml) skimmed milk
1 bay leaf
salt and pepper
8oz (227g) Shape cottage cheese
6oz (175g) wholewheat lasagne, cooked
1oz (25g) fresh wholemeal breadcrumbs
3 tbsp fresh parsley, chopped

1.   Cook the mince until well browned and drain off fat. Stir in the tomato sauce and stock. Cook gently for 3–4 minutes.

2.   Make a sauce by melting the Gold spread and stirring in the flour. Add the skimmed milk and bay leaf. Bring to the boil, stirring continuously until thickened. Remove the bay leaf, season and stir in the cottage cheese.

3.   Cover the base of an ovenproof dish with half the mince and layer with the lasagne and white sauce finishing with a topping of white sauce.

4.   Mix the breadcrumbs and parsley together and sprinkle on top. Bake for 40–45 minutes until bubbling and golden.

Serves 6. Calories per portion: 360

SLIMMERS' VEGETABLE BROTH

Make up lots of this delicious soup and freeze it for later use. It is absolutely scrumptious and very filling indeed. An ideal choice for lunch, with a crusty roll and some low-fat cheese.

4oz (100g) onions, chopped
6oz (175g) carrots, peeled and sliced
12oz (350g) swede, peeled and diced
4oz (100g) kohl rabi, peeled and diced
4oz (100g) parsnips, peeled and diced
3 cloves garlic, peeled and crushed
2 pints (1 litre) water
1 tbsp tomato purée
salt and pepper
1 tsp oregano
1 tsp thyme
3oz (75g) wholemeal macaroni
8oz (227g) Shape cottage cheese
1 tbsp fresh parsley, chopped

1.   Place all the vegetables in a large saucepan and add the water, tomato purée, seasonings and herbs. Cover and simmer for 30 minutes until tender.
2.   Add the macaroni and cook for a further 10 minutes. Add the cheese and stir into the soup with the parsley. Heat for a few minutes before serving with wholemeal rolls.

Serves 6. Calories per portion: 140

BAKED SOLE TARTARE

Using sole, this could be a smart starter for a dinner party. If you choose a cheaper white fish, like cod or coley, this is inexpensive enough for a family meal.

1 small (4oz/200g) sole (or other white fish) cleaned and skinned
5fl oz (150ml) water
1 bay leaf
3 peppercorns

5oz (150g) natural yogurt
1 egg
1 tsp capers, chopped
1 gherkin, chopped
grated zest of 1 lemon
1 tbsp parsley, chopped
salt and freshly ground black pepper

1.   Heat oven to 180°C, 350°F, gas mark 4. Place fish in a
shallow pan and add water, bay leaf and peppercorns. Bring to
the boil slowly, cover and poach for 5 minutes. Drain, place in a
shallow ovenproof dish.
2.   Beat together the yogurt and egg with the remaining ingredients. Spoon the mixture over the fish, cover and bake for 25
minutes. Serve immediately.

Serves 1. Calories per portion: 390

SPAGHETTI BOLOGNESE

*It is not spaghetti that goes to your hips, it is the sauce that goes with
it! This delicious Bolognese cuts down the fat—but you must
choose the leanest minced beef.*

1 small onion, chopped
2 cloves garlic, crushed
2 tsp dried or fresh mixed herbs
1lb (450g) lean minced beef
1 pint (575ml) beef stock
14oz (400g) chopped tomatoes
pinch of chilli powder
freshly ground black pepper
8oz (225g) wholewheat spaghetti

1.   Place onion, garlic, herbs and beef in a heavy-bottomed pan.
Heat gently, stirring all the time. Increase heat so that the meat
browns, pour off any excess fat, then add the stock, tomatoes
and seasoning. Simmer for about 40 minutes, uncovered, stirring
occasionally and adding more liquid if necessary.

2.   Meanwhile cook spaghetti in plenty of boiling salted water for 12–15 minutes when it should be cooked but still firm. Drain, arrange in a warm serving dish and pour the bolognese sauce over it.

Serves 4. Calories per portion: 400

VALERIE'S VEGETABLE HOT POT

This dish was invented by one of our slimmers, Valerie Wyatt. She says 'You can really use any vegetables at all, although I like it with the ones given in the recipe.'

12 small carrots, scraped and sliced
$^1/_2$ aubergine, unpeeled but sliced
8oz (225g) canned small white onions
$^1/_2$ small cabbage, shredded
1 small cauliflower, broken into florets
$^1/_2$ head celery, diced
5 small tomatoes, quartered
1lb (450g) potatoes, peeled and thinly sliced
2 onions, thinly sliced
2 cloves garlic, crushed
2oz (50g) low-fat spread
15fl oz (425ml) hot water
Coleman's Casserole Mix
salt and pepper

1.   Heat oven to 170°C, 325°F, gas mark 3.
2.   Place all the vegetables except the sliced onions and garlic in layers in a large casserole dish, with the sliced potatoes between each layer.
3.   Cook the onion and garlic in the low-fat spread until golden. Mix the casserole mix with the water and add to the onion mixture. Pour over the vegetables. Bake for 1½ hours or until tender.

Serves 4. Calories per portion: 280

CHICKEN AND CORN CASSEROLE

This is really easy to make and can be frozen successfully, so I've given the ingredients for a bulk cook-in. It is popular with children, who seem to adore anything with sweetcorn in it. It is so low in calories that slimmers can easily afford to add a large jacket potato and some fruit to this meal – and still have 'change' from 450 calories.

8 chicken breasts (about 6oz/175g each)
2 x 7oz (200g) cans sweetcorn, drained
2 medium onions, sliced
15oz (425g) can chopped tomatoes
1 pint (575ml) water
1 chicken stock cube
chicken seasoning
2 level tbsp cornflour
chopped parsley for garnish

1. Grill the chicken pieces for 5 minutes on each side, remove and discard skin.
2. Place sweetcorn, onions, tomatoes and juice, water, stock cube and seasoning into a large saucepan.
3. Bring to the boil and simmer for 5 minutes.
4. Blend cornflour with a little cold water and stir into the vegetable mixture.
5. Place chicken pieces in a large casserole dish and pour the sauce over. Check seasoning.
6. Cover and cook at 180°C, 350°F, gas mark 4 for 1 hour.
7. Serve, garnished with chopped parsley.

Serves: 8. Calories per portion: 240

VEGETABLES
LEEKS WITH PIQUANT YOGURT SAUCE

They grow sensational leeks up in the North of England, which is why I have included two recipes. In this one, you could use celery or even broccoli as your basic vegetable with the delicious sauce.

4 leeks
5oz (150g) natural low-fat yogurt
2 egg yolks
2 tsp lemon juice
salt and pepper
2 tsp French mustard

1. Trim leeks, then partially slit them down their length and clean in running water to remove all soil. Put into boiling, salted water and cook gently for 15–20 minutes until soft. Drain well and chill.
2. Beat yogurt, egg yolks and lemon juice together in a double boiler or in a bowl over hot water. Cook gently until thickened. Season to taste, stir in mustard and allow to cool.
3. Serve leeks sliced diagonally and topped with the sauce.

Serves 4. Calories per portion: 80

BRAISED LEEKS

You could try this recipe using whole chicory, celery or cabbage instead of leeks. Chicken or vegetable stock is best and make sure the vegetables are cooked but are still firm with bite-appeal.

12 leeks
1oz (25g) low-fat spread
$1/_2$ pint (275ml) stock
1 bay leaf
1 peppercorn
salt to taste
2 tsp cornflour

1. Trim leeks, then partially slit them down their length and clean in running water to remove all soil. Melt the low-fat spread in a shallow ovenproof dish and place the leeks on top. Cover with the stock, bay leaf, salt and peppercorns. Cook in the oven at 350°F, 180°C, gas mark 5 until tender, basting from time to time.
2. When cooked transfer leeks to a warm serving dish and put the stock in a saucepan, discarding the bay leaf and peppercorn. Blend the cornflour with a little cold water, and add to the stock.

Bring to the boil, stirring continually. Boil for 1 minute. Pour over the leeks to serve.

Serves 4. Calories per portion: 115

SWEET AND SOUR CABBAGE

Give an old favourite a new, exciting taste with this recipe. The Hermesetas Sprinkle Sweet contains only 2 calories for each spoonful and the teaspoon of oil contains just 40 calories. The recipe serves 6, so you can eat this dish as one of your 'free' vegetables with a clear conscience!

1 white cabbage, cored and shredded
1 tsp sunflower oil
2 tbsp water
2 tbsp vinegar
2 tsp Hermesetas Sprinkle Sweet
pinch of mixed spice
$1/4$ tsp salt

1.   Put the cabbage in a large pan with the rest of the ingredients. Cover and cook over a low heat for 15–20 minutes or until the cabbage is just tender but still crisp. Shake the pan often to prevent sticking.
2.   Just before serving, uncover the pan and cook quickly until all the liquid has evaporated.

Serves 6. Calories per serving: 8

SPICED CARROT AND SWEDE

Orange juice, ginger and nutmeg spice up two everyday vegetables. Again, you are adding very few calories to the basic 'free' vegetable list (swede contains just 5 calories an ounce), so you can eat plenty of this delicious and filling dish on your Fatfield diet.

4 large carrots, peeled and sliced
1lb (450g) swede, peeled and sliced
1 tsp sunflower oil
juice and grated zest of 1 orange
pinch each of ground ginger and nutmeg

1. Place carrots and swede in a shallow ovenproof dish. Combine the rest of the ingredients, and pour over.
2. Lightly cover with foil and bake in a hot oven, 190°C, 375°F, gas mark 5, for about 45 minutes or until tender.

Serves 6. Calories per serving: 55

DRESSINGS

SPICY TOMATO SAUCE

Delicious with grilled or roast chicken, fish or kebabs, this is a recipe you can make in quantity. To add bulk, include a few pulped canned tomatoes (from your 'free' vegetable list).

8fl oz (225ml) tomato juice
2fl oz (50ml) wine vinegar
1 tsp Worcestershire sauce
2oz (50g) onion, finely chopped
1 tsp dry basil
salt and freshly ground black pepper
1 tsp lemon juice
pinch of Hermesetas Sprinkle Sweet
chopped parsley to garnish

Place all the ingredients except garnish in a saucepan and bring to the boil, cover and simmer for ½ hour or until the sauce has thickened. Serve hot or cold.

Serves 4. Calories per portion: 15

FATFIELD SALAD DRESSING

3 tbsp cider vinegar
2 tbsp lemon juice
grated rind of $^1/_2$ lemon
1 tsp mixed herbs
1 clove garlic, crushed
1 tsp French mustard
salt and pepper

Place all the ingredients in a blender or screw top jar and blend well.

Serves 4. Calories per portion: 2

BARBECUE SAUCE

This is a 'must' for those summer barbecues and al fresco suppers. One Fatfield slimmer even uses it as a spread on crusty bread or in sandwiches with plenty of green salad vegetables.

$^1/_2$oz (15g) butter
1 tbsp sunflower oil
1 clove garlic, crushed
1 small onion, chopped
4 tbsp tomato ketchup
1 tbsp brown fruity sauce
1 tbsp Worcestershire sauce
1 tbsp soya sauce
1 tsp French mustard
salt and pepper
6 fl oz (175ml) hot water
$^1/_2$ beef stock cube
6oz (175g) tomatoes
2 tsp Hermesetas Sprinkle Sweet

1. Melt butter in a small pan with the oil. Add the garlic and onion and cook until soft and translucent.
2. Stir in the tomato ketchup, brown sauce, Worcestershire sauce, soya sauce and mustard. Season lightly with salt and pepper. Dissolve the stock cube in the water and add to the pan. Cover and simmer for 10 minutes.
3. Peel the tomatoes, cut in half and discard the seeds and juice. Chop the flesh and add to the pan. Simmer uncovered for 5 minutes. Purée in a blender or processor. Add the Hermesetas Sprinkle Sweet and reheat, do not boil. Serve with barbecued or grilled meat or fish.

Serves 6. Calories per portion: 65

DESSERTS

TONI'S AMAZING TRIFLE

Toni Tompsett, my assistant, is a slimmer with a young family to feed. This recipe satisfies her own sweet tooth and theirs!

1 Bird's Strawberry Sugar Free Jelly
8oz (225g) fresh or frozen strawberries
4 sponge fingers
$^1/_2$ pint (275ml) skimmed milk
1 tbsp custard powder
Hermesetas Sprinkle Sweet to taste
4 heaped tbsp Anchor Light aerosol cream

1. Break the sponge fingers into four individual bowls. Add 2oz (50g) strawberries to each, cover with $^1/_4$ of the dissolved jelly. Leave the jelly to set.
2. Mix the custard powder with 1 tbsp of cold milk. Bring the remaining milk to the boil and then pour onto the custard mixture stirring all the time. Off the heat add sweetener to taste. Leave to cool, then pour over the jelly. Add a swirl of Anchor Light aerosol cream just before serving.

Serves 4. Calories per portion: 90

APRICOT AND ORANGE MOUSSE

This is packed with goodies, and absolutely scrumptious. Make it in advance for a special occasion or a dinner party. You can keep it in the fridge for 24 hours before serving.

5oz (150g) ready-to-eat dried apricots
2 fl oz (50ml) water
7 fl oz (200ml) orange juice
1 envelope powdered gelatine
3 tbsp Hermesetas Sprinkle Sweet
7.7oz (215g) low-fat evaporated milk, chilled
1 egg white
orange peel to decorate

1. Place the apricots in a saucepan, add the water and $^3/_4$ of the orange juice. Cover and cook until tender, about 15–20 minutes. Turn into a basin and allow to cool.

2. Sprinkle the gelatine onto the remaining orange juice in a small basin and leave to soak for 10 minutes. Then stand the basin in a pan of simmering water until the gelatine has dissolved.

3. Purée the apricots and their cooking liquid in a blender or food processor. Add the dissolved gelatine and Hermesetas Sprinkle Sweet and mix well.

4. Whisk the evaporated milk until thick and foamy. Whisk the egg white until stiff. Fold the evaporated milk and egg white into the apricot mixture and then divide between 6 dishes, chill until set. Decorate with grated orange peel.

Serves 6. Calories per portion: 105

CHERRY YOGURT ICECREAM

Icecream is so easy to make that it is amazing that we don't try it more often. This recipe has to be the most delicious version of a favourite pud that I have ever tried.

15oz (425g) can black cherries
$^1/_2$ pint (275ml) Shape Double
2 x 4.4oz (125g) Shape strawberry yogurts
2 egg whites
2oz (50g) icing sugar

1. Drain the cherries and reserve the syrup. Remove all the stones.

2. Whip the Double until it holds its shape and beat in the yogurt and cherries.

3. Whisk the egg whites until stiff and fold in the icing sugar. Fold the egg-white mixture into the cherry cream. Place in a large freezer container. Freeze for about 3 hours and then beat well before completely freezing.

Serves 12. Calories per portion: 110

FRUIT BRULÉE

You can prepare this in advance and add the finishing touches before it is placed under the grill. Let your guests chat among themselves while you watch it carefully.

4oz (100g) strawberries, halved
4oz (100g) raspberries
2 tbsp blackcurrant liqueur
5fl oz (150ml) whipping cream
5fl oz (150ml) Greek yogurt
1oz (25g) golden granulated sugar

1. Mix the fruit with the liqueur in an ovenproof dish.
2. Whip the cream until it forms soft peaks, then carefully fold in the yogurt. Spoon the mixture over the fruit and smooth the surface. Cover and chill for 1 hour.
3. Sprinkle the sugar over the top. Flash under the grill until golden. Serve immediately or chill in the fridge until the topping is hard and crunchy.

Serves 4. Calories per portion: 230

JAMAICAN BANANAS

This recipe will make you feel as though you're basking on a terrace under the stars in the West Indies. Savour every spoonful slowly, for a sensual experience.

4 medium bananas, peeled
1 tbsp Hermesetas Sprinkle Sweet
$1/2$ tsp ground cinnamon
4 tbsp Bacardi
$1/2$ tsp lemon zest, finely grated
zest of $1/2$ a small orange, finely grated

1. Place each banana on a piece of foil. Cover with Sprinkle Sweet and then the cinnamon. Pour 1 tbsp Bacardi on each banana, and wrap in the foil so no juice can escape.

2. Bake in a moderate oven or on a barbecue for 5 minutes. Open and sprinkle with the zest.

Serves 4. Calories per portion: 115

GINGER SYLLABUB

This is a deliciously light dessert which is less naughty than it looks. If you have a very simple salad as a main course, you can still get up from the table feeling virtuous afterwards, having 'spent' less than 400 calories in total!

½ pt (275ml) Shape Double
grated juice and rind of ½ lemon
¼ pt (140ml) medium white wine
2oz (50g) stem ginger, finely chopped
2 egg whites
4 level tsp castor sugar
strips of lemon rind to garnish

1. Whisk Shape Double and lemon rind until soft peaks are formed. Gradually beat in lemon juice and wine, then stir in chopped ginger.
2. Whisk egg whites until stiff, then beat in the sugar and whisk until stiff again.
3. Fold into creamy mixture.
4. Spoon into serving glasses and decorate with strips of lemon rind. Serve immediately.

Serves: 6. Calories per portion: 170

ORANGE CHEESE SURPRISE

If you're a cottage cheese addict like me, you'll love this pudding. The orange juice and liqueur give the cheese a lovely tangy flavour, and the rolled oats provide crunch-appeal. It's surprisingly filling, so eat it after a very light main course.

4 large oranges
1 tbsp orange liqueur
4oz (100g) black grapes, halved and seeded

156

8oz (225g) low-fat cottage cheese
4 tbsp rolled oats, toasted

1. Cut a thin slice from the base of each orange so it stands up in an individual sundae dish.
2. Cut the top one-third from each orange and scoop out all the flesh. Reserve the 'hats' for decoration.
3. Chop the flesh and put into a bowl with the liqueur and grapes. Cover and chill for a few hours or overnight.
4. Put the cottage cheese into a bowl, stir in the toasted oats and the fruit mixture.
5. Pile into the orange shells and replace 'hats'.

Serves: 4. Calories per portion: 180

NUTTY BAKED APPLES WITH MANGO SAUCE
This pudding is elegant enough for a dinner party but it would also make a delicious lunchtime main course dish. The sauce is absolutely yummy with icecream too.

2 cooking apples
1 egg, size 4 or 5, beaten
3fl oz (75ml) natural low-fat yogurt
½oz (15g) castor sugar
juice of ½ lemon
2oz (50g) Edam, finely grated
1 level tbsp coarsely chopped walnuts
2 level tbsp raisins
pinch of cinnamon
sprigs of mint for decoration

Sauce
1 mango
½ tsp lemon juice
1 tsp Hermesetas granulated sweetener

1.   Cut the apples in half and remove the core. Using a pointed spoon, carefully hollow out about half of the apple. Cut flesh into small pieces.
2.   Pre-heat oven to 150°C, 300°F, gas mark 2.

3.   Mix beaten egg in a bowl with the chopped apple and other main ingredients.

4.   Fill the hollowed-out apples with this mixture.

5.   Place in an ovenproof dish and cook in a preheated oven for 30 minutes, until the filling is firm.

6.   Allow to cool while you make the sauce.

7.   Stone and peel the mango and cut the flesh into pieces.

8.   Mix with the lemon juice and granulated sweetener and purée in a blender or press through a fine sieve.

9.   Spoon the sauce onto 4 dessert plates and place the filled, cooled apples in the centre. Decorate with mint sprigs and serve immediately.

Serves: 4. Calories per portion: 170 (sauce alone: 30)

FATFIELD FAVOURITES

Here is a list of branded foods and drinks which our Fatfield slimmers have found especially helpful and delicious on the diet:

FOOD	PORTION	CALORIES
Breakfast Cereals		
Kellogg's Sultana Bran	1oz (25g)	91
Kellogg's Fruit 'n Fibre	1oz (25g)	102
Shredded Wheat	1	80
Weetabix	1	65
Crispbreads		
High Fibre Ryvita	1 slice	21
Crackerbread	1 slice	20
Cereal Bars		
Quaker Harvest Crunch, Raisin	1	80
Granose Fruit Snack Bar, Apricot, Fig or Prune	1	80
Dairy Products		
Boots Shapers Yogurts	5oz (125g) pot	60
Delight Low Fat Cheese Spread portions	1	35
Delight Low Fat Soft Cheese with Garlic and Herbs	1oz (25g)	41
Delight Very Low Fat Spread	1oz (25g)	64
St Ivel Shape Cottage Cheese, Italian, Mexican, Natural or Pineapple	4oz (113g) pot	80
St Ivel Shape yogurts	5oz (125g) pot	60

St Ivel Shape Fromage Frais	4oz (100g) pot	50
Tesco Half Fat Cheddar	1oz (25g)	74

Sweeteners

Hermesetas Light or Sprinkle Sweet	1 level tsp (5ml)	2

Ready Meals

Bird's Eye Menu Master:		
Beef in Stout with Herb Dumplings	1 pack	215
Creamy Chicken and Broccoli Bake	1 pack	235
Somerset Chicken in Cider	1 pack	200
Boots Shapers Frozen Recipe Dishes:		
Beef Lasagne or Salmon Mornay	1 pack	300
Vegetable Gratin	1 pack	290
Findus Lean Cuisine:		
Chicken a l'orange with Almond Rice	1 pack	275
Kashmir Chicken Curry or Lamb Tikka Masala	1 pack	295
Fisherman's Pie or Prawn Curry with Rice	1 pack	275
Findus Lean Cuisine for Healthy Appetites:		
Farmhouse Chicken Casserole with Vegetables	1 pack	335
Sainsbury's:		
Chicken Korma with Turmeric Rice	1 pack	270
St Michael Chilled Meals:		
Chilli Con Carne	1 pack	275

FATFIELD FAVOURITES

Snacks and Salads

Golden Wonder Pot Pasta Bolognaise	1 pot	245
Boots Shapers Pot Meal, Beef Chow Mein	1 pot	155
St Ivel Shape coleslaw	5½oz (142g) pot	130
Tesco Healthy Eating Low Calorie Potato Salad	10oz (250g)	250

Drinks

Ovaltine Options, all flavours	1 cup	40
Instant Bovril	1 sachet	20
Sainsbury's Reduced Calorie Exotic Fruit Juice	¼ pt	20
Barbican Low Alcohol Lager	275ml bottle	45
Danish Light Low Alcohol Lager	320ml can	55
Jung's De-Alcoholized Extra Dry White Wine	5fl oz (142ml)	10

Puddings

Ambrosia Pot Low Fat Rice Pudding	1 pot	115
Bird's Sugar Free Jelly	1 pack	50
Ross Mousse, all flavours	1 pot	90
Tesco Healthy Eating Dessert, Blackcurrant flavour	1 pack	65

Soups

Batchelors Slim a Soups, all flavours	1 sachet	40
Batchelors Slim a Soup Specials, all flavours	1 sachet	60

WHAT SHOULD YOU WEIGH?

Don't aim too low when you are deciding
on your goal weight. As I have said before, the best weight for
you is the one at which you feel and look good. It may well be
that a certain amount of plumpness suits you!
Below is a chart for recording your weekly weight-loss.
Weigh in on the same scales, at the same time of day. Measure
your chest, waist, and hips at the same time – and don't cheat
by pulling your tape-measure in too tightly.

DATE	WEIGHT	BUST	WAIST	HIPS

YOUR FOOD DIARY

During the first, difficult weeks of your diet, it is a good idea to keep a food diary. Note *exactly* what you ate, and how you felt when you ate it. If you cheated, you must include all the naughty nibbles and drinks which were not on your official Fatfield food plan.

Every week, sit down quietly, and go through the diary. Try to plan a strategy for dealing with difficult moments that crop up again and again. For instance, if you always seem to nibble bread and butter when you are cutting sandwiches for your childrens' tea, make sure you have a mug of slimmer's soup handy to sip instead.

If you habitually go astray when the 11am snack trolley comes round the office, make sure you are *out* of the room at that time or have some fresh fruit in your desk to eat instead of a fattening snack.

Make yourself a diary like this, and keep it daily:

	Breakfast	Lunch	Supper	Drinks and Nibbles
MONDAY				
Place	ON THE BUS	AT WORK	AT HOME	THE PUB
Time	8.30AM	1PM	6PM	9PM
What I ate	BAG OF SWEETS	WHOLEMEAL SANDWICH FRUIT	FATFIELD SHEPHERD'S PIE	GIN & TONIC PORK PIE
How I felt	CROSS WITH MYSELF!	VIRTUOUS!	FULL UP!	A BIT DOWN (SHOULD HAVE EATEN A BETTER BREAKFAST!)

SIGN ON AND
SLIM DOWN

One of the best ways to motivate yourself to lose weight, is to make a pact with the one person who will be affected most by your success or failure – *you!*

As I explained in Chapter Seven, it is a good idea to sign some kind of pledge which you can keep safely – perhaps pinned on the kitchen wall – until you have lost weight. Or, get someone such as your partner, your doctor (or even *me!*) to keep it safely for you.

We have a special Fatfield Charter (*see* opposite), which we ask our slimmers to fill in before they start our diet. The simple act of writing down your aims will start you off on the correct footing for successful slimming.

If you want to send your completed Charter to me, include details of your weight problems, plus a polaroid photograph. Include your full name and address and daytime telephone number.

When you reach the targets set out in your Charter, send me another Polaroid picture, with details of your achievement. I will return the Charter to you, endorsed with the Fatfield Seal of Excellence!

The address is: Fatfield Charter, Sally Ann Voak, PO Box 618, Coulsdon, Surrey CR5 1RU

THE FATFIELD CHARTER

I, ... , promise to follow the Fatfield Diet faithfully and diligently until I lose a total of . . . . lb in weight.

I aim to reach that target on . . . . (date)

Forsaking all other diets, I will remain true to the Fatfield principles of eating large, healthy meals.

I will try not to cheat, but if I do fall by the wayside I will not feel guilty. Instead, I will pull myself together and make up for my transgressions on the following day!

I will also endeavour to take more exercise. This is an outline of my exercise plan . . . .
. . . .
. . . .

When I have lost 7lb I promise that I will give myself a present or treat, such as . . . .

When I have lost 1 stone, I promise that I will give myself a more expensive gift or larger treat, such as
. . . .

When I reach my goal weight, I will buy myself something very special indeed, such as . . . .
. . . .

Signed this day . . . . (date),

in the presence of

Witness No. One . . . . (signature)

Witness No. Two . . . . (signature)